DISABILITY AND POPULAR CULTURE

The Cultural Politics of Media and Popular Culture

Series Editor:
C. Richard King
Washington State University, USA

Dedicated to a renewed engagement with culture, this series fosters critical, contextual analyses and cross-disciplinary examinations of popular culture as a site of cultural politics. It welcomes theoretically grounded and critically engaged accounts of the politics of contemporary popular culture and the popular dimensions of cultural politics. Without being aligned to a specific theoretical or methodological approach, *The Cultural Politics of Media and Popular Culture* publishes monographs and edited collections that promote dialogues on central subjects, such as representation, identity, power, consumption, citizenship, desire and difference.

Offering approachable and insightful analyses that complicate race, class, gender, sexuality, (dis)ability and nation across various sites of production and consumption, including film, television, music, advertising, sport, fashion, food, youth, subcultures and new media, *The Cultural Politics of Media and Popular Culture* welcomes work that explores the importance of text, context and subtext as these relate to the ways in which popular culture works alongside hegemony.

Also available in the series

Beyond Hate
White Power and Popular Culture
C. Richard King and David J. Leonard
ISBN: 978-1-4724-2746-5

The American Imperial Gothic
Popular Culture, Empire, Violence
Johan Höglund
ISBN: 978-1-4094-4954-6

Representations of HIV/AIDS in Contemporary Hispano-American and Caribbean Culture
Cuerpos suiSIDAs
Gustavo Subero
ISBN: 978-1-4724-2595-9

Disability, Obesity and Ageing
Popular Media Identifications
Debbie Rodan, Katie Ellis and Pia Lebeck
ISBN: 978-1-4094-4051-2

Disability and Popular Culture

Focusing Passion,

Creating Community and Expressing Defiance

KATIE ELLIS
Curtin University, Australia

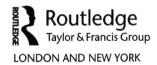

Routledge
Taylor & Francis Group

LONDON AND NEW YORK

First published 2015 by Ashgate Publishing

2 Park Square, Milton Park, Abingdon, Oxfordshire OX14 4RN
52 Vanderbilt Avenue, New York, NY 10017

Routledge is an imprint of the Taylor & Francis Group, an informa business

First issued in paperback 2020

British Library Cataloguing in Publication Data
A catalogue record for this book is available from the British Library.

The Library of Congress has cataloged the printed edition as follows:
Ellis, Katie, 1978-
  Disability and popular culture : focusing passion, creating community and expressing defiance
/ by Katie Ellis.
    pages cm. -- (The cultural politics of media and popular culture)
  Includes bibliographical references and index.
  ISBN 978-1-4724-1178-5 (hardback)
  1. People with disabilities in mass media. 2. Popular culture. I. Title.
  HV1568.E445 2015

                                                                    2014030616

ISBN 978-1-4724-1178-5 (hbk)
ISBN 978-0-367-66900-3 (pbk)

Contents

For my partners in pop, Amanda, Leanne and the Barbies, books, music, movies and the TV shows we were and weren't allowed to watch!

List of Figures and Tables

Figures

Tables

Acknowledgements

Discovering the social model of disability was a threshold moment in my personal and academic life. The idea that society created the problem of disability through inaccessible environments and discriminatory attitudes was simply revolutionary to me. So I thank those 1970s British activists for their insight, activism and 'big idea' *and* the theorists who later developed the cultural model for developing a way to think, talk and theorise about these things.

I see the continuing relevance of the social model of disability but also its inability to explain every situation. In this book I look at disability through the lens of popular culture and popular culture through the lens of disability. This study in part grew out of my frustrations with the social model, for not recognising the pleasures of popular culture or the changes in the ways disability has figured throughout popular culture. The ways people use popular culture to mark out community and play with identities. Several of the texts I analyse in this book are my own pop culture favourites which have in some way spoken to me on my journey through disability and impairment; others are significant moments in contemporary popular culture that have been singled out for discussion within the disability community and, while I may not have begun my research as a fan of these texts, I have come to respect them and indeed recognise them as important battle grounds in the ongoing fight for disability inclusion. I thank the creators of popular culture for their embrace of disability and the people with disability who use these texts in their own lives, in their own ways.

I have enjoyed writing this book; it has been a fantastic opportunity to engage with popular culture, the exciting new wave of television and web programming in particular and to (re)discover some popular culture that didn't speak to me in its heyday. I love popular culture; I cry at movies and once I start laughing can find it difficult to stop. I fully embrace the journey of television characters and often seek out more information about them online. I thank everyone, the students, colleagues and friends, who have shared their opinions about disability and popular culture with me but especially my sisters Amanda and Leanne for being switched on, critical and avid consumers of popular culture. To our parents George and Carleen thank you for instilling an important affirmative ethics of popular culture critique and enjoyment.

Many people have read or heard pieces of this book and generously gave of their time to discuss ideas with me: Kai-Ti Kao, Lauren O'Mahony, Pia Lebeck, Gerard Goggin, Beth Haller, Matt Harrison, Mick Broderick, Mike Kent, Susan

Leong, Carleen Ellis and Tara Brabazon. I also thank the anonymous readers of this book who have offered insightful and encouraging feedback at every stage. Chris Pearce, my partner in life and in watching *Breaking Bad*, your support makes this book, and everything else, possible. Stella, my littlest consumer of pop, I have learnt so much with and from you and have been pleasantly surprised to discover the presence of disability throughout children's popular culture, toys, television and even in toddler bop!

Thanks are also due to Neil Jordan at Ashgate Publishing for taking an interest in this project and for shepherding it through the publication process and to C. Richard King the editor of *The Cultural Politics of Media and Popular Culture* series that I am privileged to be a part of. Vital research assistance was provided by Melissa Merchant and I thank Christine Brewer and Ceri Clocherty for helping to prepare the final manuscript for publication. Thank you also to Curtin University and the School of Media Communication and Creative Arts for providing a Publications grant to complete the manuscript. I am also grateful to the Australian Research Council for the privilege of a Discovery Early Career Research Award (DE130101712) on *Disability and Digital Television*, of which this book is an output.

Chapter 1
Introduction: Producerly Disability

In November 2010 Steve Tucker, a public servant working in the Australian Capital Territory, sent an email to 7,000 of his government department co-workers trying to track down a woman he'd met on a night out with colleagues. The email read in part:

> She left a strong and positive impression on me. Unfortunately, people got in the way after we met and I didn't get to finish our meeting how I wanted to. This has been bugging me ever since. If you can kindly let [her] know that I would like to get in contact with her or alternatively get in touch with myself, I will be very appreciative. (Tucker cited in johnboy, 2010)

He concluded the email with the assertion that 'life is too short for regret'. As Australians sighed a collective 'what a sleaze', we thought we had him all figured out. Tucker was compared to Napoléon, Romeo, and Patrick Moberg, the 21-year-old who enlisted the help of the blogosphere in 2007 to track down a girl he was too shy to talk to on the train. We rolled our eyes at Tucker's attempt to locate the 'tall and olive skinned [Olivia]' while the email was forwarded on to a further 22 million people. So close to Christmas, it was a slow news week and, as Tucker's motives were voraciously debated around water coolers, on breakfast television and in the comments section of online newspapers, he went into hiding.

Then, just as the story was all but dead, Tucker emailed journalist and blogger Sam de Brito to tell 'his side'. His side changed everything. Steve Tucker, wasn't just *some guy*, he had cerebral palsy – he was disabled. His response to the media attention detailed experiences of bullying, teenaged angst, early 20s' uncertainty, romantic rejection, self-sabotage and a more recent state of awareness and insight. He was trying to track down Olivia as part of a broader project on himself and how he approached life. The email he sent to his colleagues was not about 'picking up' it was about social constructions of life, gender and disability:

> … about people dealing with disability; those who cannot communicate their suffering and the families that care for these people tirelessly. It is about telling peer pressure to go f--- itself. It's childish behaviour and it impacts our adult lives in ways we don't see. It is about gender stereotypes (both of them) and social conditioning. It is about mental health and getting help if needed. It is about

telling people what they mean to us while life is good. Not when a personal crisis hits. Tomorrow isn't a guarantee for any of us. It is about standing up to society and illustrating that it has lost its way. We live in a culture of fear. Society had dimmed my spirit for long enough. (Tucker cited in de Brito, 2010)

This was a media-literate response. Tucker evaluated both the media narrative around his email as well as, further back, towards representations of masculinity and disability in general to produce a new critique. While his focus on internalising and overcoming socially disabling pressures could be read as further evidence of the individualisation of disability, he provided a perspective on disability as subject to social and cultural pressures that was unique to Australian media and culture.

Like race, class, gender and sexuality, disability is a pervasive image in media and popular culture and a provocative topic among philosophers, theorists, academics and bloggers. *Disability and Popular Culture* attends to the dominance of images of disability in popular culture as a site of cultural politics. This book covers a broad range of subjects, texts, and concerns that lie at the intersection of disability and cultural studies, including media representation, identity, the beauty myth, aesthetics, ableism, new media, children's toys and sport.

Disability, Society and Culture

While, for many, disability can be explained in a straightforward way using medical discourses, critical disability theorists recognise that disability is both socially and culturally constructed. Social and cultural models of disability have emerged in response to the dominating medicalisation of disability as a personal problem to overcome. Critical approaches to disability are often described as emerging concurrently on either side of the Atlantic, in the UK and US, each with slightly different focus. Whereas the UK model leveraged that country's tradition of the labour movement and focused on issues related to employment, the US critical disability approach was heavily influenced by gains made within civil rights.

The Social Model

To begin in the UK, the field is dominated by the 'social model of disability'. This model sees disability as the restriction of social activity imposed on top of people that have impairments and is very much concerned with access to the workforce. Prominent UK social model activist Vic Finkelstein (1981) proposed three stages of disability which were closely tied to the employment possibilities of particular epochs. The first stage of disability occurred during the feudal era where people with disability worked within and were cared for by the family unit. Hand-built machinery could be modified to suit variations in bodies and adaptive technology was not unusual. Then, with the advent of the industrial revolution, the concept of able-bodied normality was established as work expectations shifted towards interchangeable bodies who could come in and out of the production line without need for variation in machinery. It was during the second stage that disability was medicalised as institutions caring for the disabled and insane were established and people with disability were removed from public view and placed into these institutions. Finally, Finkelstein proposed a third stage of disability where new information technologies would allow the disabled to re-enter the workforce, again through the use of adaptive technologies.

The social model of disability has been integral in raising awareness of disability as subject to socially created oppression; however, it has also been accused of neglecting cultural imagery, certain personal experiences and the impacts of impairment. The social model proposed a clear distinction between disability as a form of socially created oppression and impairment as existing in the body, and also binarised the distinction between the medical model and social model of disability. As Tom Shakespeare (2006) argues, a number of critiques of disability (more than I am able to fully elaborate on in this brief introduction) which proceeded from a social oppression framework emerged around the same time as the social model but did not necessarily insist on these overt political distinctions. Many of these approaches recognise the relevance of impairment while still foregrounding disability as a subject to social-contextual factors.

The Cultural Model

US critical theorists David Mitchell and Sharon Snyder (2006) proposed a 'cultural model of disability' in an attempt to 'incorporate both the outer and inner reaches of culture and experience as a combination of profoundly social and biological forces' (p. 7). They saw disability as an intricate 'phenomenological value that is not purely synonymous with the process of social disablement' (p. 6). Although the strict distinction between disability and impairment is not overt within US cultural models of disability, 'the overarching orientation is social and cultural, not medical or individualist' (Shakespeare, 2006, p. 25).

Mitchell and Snyder (2000) outline the ways cultural representations of disability have been approached by disability theorists to identify a progression of analysis through a number of areas of focus. In a similar fashion to many identity based areas of enquiry, cultural analysis began with the recognition of stereotypes. For Mitchel and Snyder this approach can be divided into 'negative imagery' which identifies and categorises damaging reoccurring stereotypes of disability and 'social realist' approaches designed to counter these caricatures of disability which are considered to be 'inaccurate and misleading' (p. 21). Their next two categories – 'new historicism' and 'biographical criticism' – also work in concert. New historicism recognises that images of disability emerge in the context of particular eras and cultures. In this way, positive and negative imagery comes to be understood as context-specific and always in a process of construction. Authors with disability have been actively sought out by disability theorists as part of this historical revisionism. A number of disabled, deformed and ill authors have been identified and their works interrogated for what they reveal about the relationship between literature and medicine for example. Finally, 'transgressive reappropriation' recognises the potential for cultural subversion in images of disability which may be considered negative. They recommend critical theorists undertake a consideration of how disability works as a narrative prosthesis in popular media and culture. For Mitchell and Snyder, a 'narrative prosthetics' functions as:

> ... a character-making trope in the writer's arsenal, as a social category of deviance, as a symbolic vehicle for meaning-making and cultural critique, and as an option in the narrative negotiation of disabled subjectivity. (Snyder and Mitchell, 2000, p. 1)

It is clear that disability functioned as a narrative prosthesis – or a prop to structure and support the story – in the Steve Tucker story. Whereas initially Tucker was framed as an overly enthusiastic young man enjoying the night life and abusing his workplace email system, once he revealed the disability connection he became an inspirational young man triumphing over adversary. His response also leveraged this common cultural narrative (prosthesis) to shift perceptions. The disability connection gave this story depth and meaning and took the 'life is too short' mantra to another level. It also troubled our initial interpretation and broader cultural understanding of masculinity, disability, how we treat other people, and the media's quick rush to judgement.

Rosemarie Garland-Thomson offers a particularly useful framework for understanding disability that I will draw on throughout this book:

> Disability has four aspects: first, it is a system for interpreting bodily variations; second, it is a relation between bodies and their environments; third, it is a set of practices that produce both the able-bodied and the disabled; fourth, it is a way of describing the inherent instability of the embodied self. (Garland-Thomson, 2002, p. 74)

The experience of disability is therefore shaped by social and cultural factors. However, despite Mitchell and Snyder's observations, it is often claimed that the

4

image of disability in media and culture has not changed (see Darke, 2004; Gerber, 2012; Longmore, 1987). Yet, a number of social and cultural changes have taken place to improve the social position of people with disability since disability in media and culture came to the attention of disability academics and activists. For example, throughout the 1990s, changes in legislation on an international scale were attempting to make society a more equitable place for people with disability. An emerging disability rights movement challenged the idea that disability was an individual's problem and forced a disabling society to take some responsibility. As a result of the politicisation of disability and the emergence of a disability culture movement, the image of disability in popular culture began to change during the 1990s and 2000s. Where previously disability was used as an exit strategy to kill off characters in soap operas, there are now permanent characters and cast members with disability. Due to the success of the Paralympics Games (and the popularity of the documentary film *Murderball*), disabled sports are becoming mainstream. Other important developments include the introduction of children's toys that have disabilities to the mainstream toy market and the inclusion of disability in magazine and music video discourses of beauty.

The *Game of Thrones* character Tyrion Lannister has some particularly useful observations that derive from both social and cultural models of disability and reflect changing attitudes around disability oppression and inclusion in popular culture. As a dwarf, Tyrion faces prejudice from the society in which he lives and is constantly devalued by his father, Tywin, who resents him for his disability and his mother's death in childbirth. Tywin describes wanting to carry Tyrion into the sea and 'let the waves wash [him] away', variously calling him a 'stunted fool', and 'an ill-made, spiteful little creature full of envy, lust, and low cunning'. Although Tywin constantly reminds Tyrion of his socially devalued qualities, Tyrion displays intellect, compassion, loyalty, bravery and wit. His compassion extends to rival family the Starks as he encourages second son Bran to use modified stirrups to ride a horse after he acquires a spinal injury. He also offers illegitimate son Jon Snow advice on how to deal with other people's prejudice: 'Let me give you some advice, bastard: Never forget what you are. The rest of the world will not. Wear it like armour, and it can never be used to hurt you.' As Tyrion explains that 'all dwarves are bastards in their father's eyes', his encouragement of Jon Snow becomes a statement about disability rights and inclusion that although set in another time and place has clear resonance today. *Game of Thrones* features a number of characters with disability and develops them as complex people with strengths *and* weaknesses.

Throughout this book I seek to bring together social and cultural models of disability to explore the presence of disability in popular culture and consider the ways popular culture reflects social change, debates pertinent issues and, indeed, is pleasurable. As I discuss throughout this book, disability features prominently in popular culture, including in film, television, toys, sport, advertising, and music video, as a central cultural identity and category. Sometimes, as is commonly the case with *Game of Thrones*, the disability relevance is overlooked, even while clear and direct statements are made about disability inclusion.

In their landmark collection of essays on popular culture *Hop on Pop*, Henry Jenkins, Tara McPherson and Jane Shattac (2002) observe that one of the challenges in engaging with popular culture for populations who have historically been excluded from production and representation is the question of how to 'acknowledge the pleasures they have derived from engaging with popular culture as well as their rage and frustration about its silences, exclusions and assaults on their lives' (p. 10). This is a useful starting point for thinking about disability and popular culture because, as the social model recognises, people with disabilities have been excluded from production and representation (see Barnes, 1992; Darke, 2004; Hevey, 1992), yet research and even online activity suggests people with disabilities gain pleasure from popular culture. These pleasures open a space for critical engagement. As popular culture and popular memory theorist Tara Brabazon maintains, popular culture offers people a sense of identity and group cohesion:

> Popular culture allows audiences to make sense of their lives, when the structures and truths of families, governments and the workplace contradict experiences. Film, television and popular music have a transformative impact on cultural groups, creating enthusiastic audiences who are able to mark out and claim their differences. (Brabazon, 2004, p. 21)

Brabazon's observations emerge from a particular tradition of the study of popular culture, a framework that has not been embraced by some sectors of critical disability studies.

Popular Culture

At the same time that the concept of able-bodied normality was being established in the second phase of disability, the same cultural shift impacted on the creation and interpretation of popular culture when class distinctions emerged through the 'new work relations of industrial capitalism' (Storey, 2003, p. 16). As a result, a clear distinction emerged between popular culture produced for and enjoyed by the masses, and high culture as 'the best that has been thought and known in the world' (Arnold, 2006, p. xxii). In simple terms, this is a division between high art and popular culture, a division still operating today.

The Marxist-inspired Frankfurt School of cultural studies proceeded from this line of enquiry. Notably, intellectuals Theodor Adorno and Max Horkheimer (1972) are scathing in their assessment of popular culture as 'business' and 'not art'. They rejected the notion that people spontaneously choose culture. Instead, they argue that culture is an industry which employs capitalist means of coercion to manipulate people into continually consuming. Adorno and Horkheimer (1972) claim that popular culture, through its appeal to the masses, creates cultural dupes and citizens who become re-enslaved to the ideology of capitalism through their dependence on it. They argue that the 'absolute power of capitalism' (p. 120) is stamped onto magazines, films, radio, even architecture. The audience is coerced into insisting that the same ideology which enslaves them is constantly reproduced, a practice with which producers are happy to oblige.

This discussion reveals the ways popular culture is regarded as both inferior to high culture and as the originator of a number of social problems. In short, the audience is considered passive and the solution is to value elite forms of art as culturally superior. This is a position that has been taken up by several disability theorists who proceed from a social model perspective. For example, in his seminal book *The Politics of Disablement*, Michael Oliver (1990) argued people with disability are never presented as ordinary people with ordinary problems in popular culture, always emerging as superheroes, villains or tragic individuals. Sheila Riddell and Nick Watson (2003) use Oliver's 1990 observation to reject criticisms that the social model has not adequately engaged with culture and cultural theorists. They posit that the social model's unwillingness to draw on cultural studies – with its more recent focus on active audiences and shifting identities – was related to connections Oliver identified between cultural imagery which individualised and medicalised disability, and a similar focus he saw operating in 'the professions' and which he highlighted in his early work (see Oliver, 1990; Riddell and Watson, 2003).

However, recognition of the impact of cultural imagery and narratives has gradually increased from a disability perspective. As discussed, analysis began with the recognition of stereotypes. For example Barnes, Mercer and Shakespeare (1999) see the representation of disability and what it means to be disabled as being communicated through damaging stereotypes. The processes of producing meanings of normality mean disabled people are 'different'. Like Oliver, Barnes et al.'s (1999) comment that people with disability are most often represented as not powerful, nor attractive, or their impairment is a metaphor for evil.

Positive versus Negative Stereotypes

The idea of positive versus negative stereotypes of disability has been discussed within the social model of disability and similarly within media guidelines. However, as critics have pointed out, positive stereotypes are equally as constructed as negative stereotypes and are, in fact, context-specific. What is considered positive in one area or discipline of thought may not be considered positive in another. As Mitchell and Snyder (2006) argue, representations are inevitably 'bound to their own historical moment's shortcomings, idiosyncrasies, and obsessions' (p. 201). Instead of dividing the representation of disability into a positive and negative binary opposition, it is important that we see people with disability along the full spectrum of human experience and popular culture characterisation – as good, bad, right, wrong, strong and weak. There needs to be moments where disability is relevant and irrelevant.

Games of Thrones – which was awarded a Media Access Award in 2013 in recognition of its efforts in 'promoting awareness of the disability experience, accessibility for people with disabilities, and the accurate depiction of characters with disabilities' (*Winter Is Coming*, 2013) – includes a number of characters with disability (both acquired and lifelong). While these characters may be superheroes, villains or tragic individuals, the narrative frequently speaks to the social disablement of people who have impairments. Although within the fantasy genre, this cult TV show reflects current values regarding disability and has been recognised as speaking to the contemporary disability experience:

> Since its earliest episodes, [Game of Thrones] has introduced us to a paralyzed boy with a supernatural gift, has endeared us to a Little Person defined not by his height but by his wit, and has regularly mined the lives of "cripples, bastards, and broken things" to celebrate their strengths and complexities. In fact, it is a fantastic credit … that Game of Thrones is not commonly thought of as a show that "deals with" disability – it is something even better: a show that embraces the reality that no one is easily definable. (David Radcliff cited in *Winter Is Coming*, 2013)

Following the announcement of this award, a number of people with and without disability discussed their interpretation of *Game of Thrones* in the context of their lives and experiences. Viewers active on the *Winter is Coming* blog discussed the plethora of minor characters with disability, the tendency to 'label' people with disability, and the ways *Game of Thrones* innovated both the fantasy genre and the overall cultural representation of people with disabilities. Tyrion in particular is a favourite character, as That Stark boy comments:

> I began to love the series because of Tyrion, I was just fucking tired of seeing dwarves as clowns in every goddamned show I watched – and hear everyone around me applauding – and when I saw that dwarf that was just as complex as any other character I knew this show was just as badass as they said. (That Stark boy comment on *Winter Is Coming*, 2013)

Game of Thrones is an example of popular culture that creates community and brings people together. Raymond Williams' 1958 argument that culture was 'ordinary' represented a seismic shift in cultural studies and has been heralded with establishing the discipline (Jenkins et al., 2002). While he held some sympathy for the view that certain forms of culture were superior, for Williams, culture joined people together in a community (Brantlinger, 1991). Similarly, John Fiske argued for a reconceptualisation of popular culture away from the consumption of images towards a 'productive process'. He urged theorists to shift their thinking away from the disciplinary power of texts and what 'the people' are reading towards 'how' they are reading it (Fiske, 1989, 2010, p. 112). While we should remain aware and critical of the ways the dominant ideology is reflected and reinforced in popular culture, there is still room for optimism in the ways people counter these top down strategies with bottom up activities, active audience insights and textual poaching. However, disability remains an under explored area in this regard and continues to be marginalised within identity based analysis.

The Real Limitation from Which to Escape

As Mitchell and Snyder (2000) note, disability does not fit neatly into a discourse of marginalisation despite its similarity to other identity based areas of inquiry such as gender, race or sexuality. While it is well recognised that social factors contribute to the creation and experience of people fitting into these groups, disability has traditionally remained outside questions of discourse, culture, communication and meaning.

This tension was actually explored in an episode of the hit 1990s postfeminist television comedy drama *Ally McBeal* when Ally's old college classmate, now boss, Richard Fish attempts to make the argument in court that women are disabled by society's expectations of them. A clever argument that articulates notions of social disablement and draws a connection between people with disabilities and women as subjugated groups, the premise is hotly rejected by female members of the firm – Ally and Georgia in particular. Yet Richard is not discouraged, leading to one of his famous Fishisms (unique way of looking at the world articulated in a witty and borderline nonsensical way):

> Georgia, give me your shoe. Why would a grown person wear these? They are hugely uncomfortable, make it easier to fall, cause back problems, but, hey – call it fashion. What kind of person would spend an equivalent of two years painting her face and plucking out her eyebrows, and putting silicone or saline in her chest? There is a name for this kind of person, "woman". Why? Because, we "men" like it. Don't talk to me about equality. Don't tell me you aren't disabled. (The Playing Field S1 E18)

9

Richard is not arguing that there is an intrinsic reason why women behave and dress in this way – the cause is not biological. In fact, Richard acknowledges that women are socially pressured to perform these rituals. Ally and Georgia, on the other hand, flatly refuse any identification with people with disability, finding it to be a disempowering notion. Feminist criticism of this episode has also found the connection between disability and gender to be problematic, outrageous even (Zeisler, 2008). It is intriguing, however, that Zeisler (2008) describes the association between disability and female subjugation as an example of a 'cheap and mean-spirited [shot] at feminism and female capability' (p. 98).

Disability journalist and co-founder of the US disability lifestyle magazine and multimedia group *We*, Charles A. Riley III (2005), is critical of the symbolic use of disability throughout *Ally McBeal*. He argues that most of the jokes were 'at the expense of people with disabilities, including obsessive-compulsive disorder and stuttering' (p. 94) and that this became increasingly problematic as the stars on the show began experiencing their own medical problems off screen in their personal lives. For Riley, *Ally McBeal* tiptoed 'along a razor's edge between sophisticated disability-awareness and flagrant insults to keep the laughs going' (p. 95). His critique makes clear connections to freak shows, a cultural form that has plagued the representation of disability but also identifies the current state of play of disability and popular culture – a razor's edge between disability awareness and the same old subjugation. In short, critical discourses of disability are articulated in constant tension with the dominant ableist ideology.

The Producerly Text

John Fiske identifies this tension as an important feature in turning mass-produced culture into *popular* culture. He draws on Barthes distinction between the readerly and writerly text to add a third category which encompasses popular culture – the producerly text. Readerly texts are more popular and invite passive consumption with a relatively fixed process of meaning making, while the writerly text 'challenges the reader to constantly rewrite it, to make sense out of it'. Writerly texts encourage readers to 'participate in the construction of meaning' (Fiske, 1989, 2010, p. 83). Cultural disability theorists and practitioners in performance related fields have established the political potential of disability texts and performances which encourage their audience to participate in the construction of meaning (see Sandahl and Auslander, 2005). For Barthes, writerly texts exist in the realm of avant-garde. Fiske, however, maintains that his third category 'producerly' describes the popular writerly text. While preferred meanings can be accommodated, so can those which expose and question these meanings. Producerly popular texts are progressive:

[The producerly text] offers itself up to popular production; it exposes, however reluctantly, the vulnerabilities, limitations, and weaknesses of its preferred meanings; it contains, while attempting to repress them, voices that contradict the ones it prefers; it has loose ends that escape its control, its meanings exceed its own power to discipline them, its gaps are wide enough for whole new texts to be produced in them – it is, in a very real sense, beyond its own control. (Fiske, 1989, 2010, p. 83)

I explore producerly texts which offer a representation of disability throughout this book. These texts can be considered simultaneously disabling and enabling. On one level these texts could be interpreted as readerly, or inviting a passive acceptance of the domination of people with disabilities. Yet they offer the possibility of thinking differently about ourselves, of creating new concepts and developing a critical theory which recognises what Rosi Braidolli (2010) calls 'affirmative ethics'. For Braidolli critical theory must critique *and* offer positive alternatives.

Resistance and Incorporation

Throughout this book, I approach audiences, viewers and consumers as active in the choices they make and the meanings they gain from media and popular culture, arguing that moments of resistance are possible even in popular culture that adopt an ableist tone. This argument follows the work of John Fiske who noted the way young girls interpreted Madonna as a strong female role model who could be controlled by no man despite her obvious construction as a 'sex symbol'. He also reflected on the ways female viewers of *Charlie's Angels* 'poached' or selected only the feminist moments of the text to pay attention to and did not watch the end of the show when patriarchal authority was re-established through Charlie's paternalistic praise. However, as E. Graham McKinley (1997) argues in a study of the television program *Beverly Hills 90210*, resistance takes *work*. The result is that a large number of the audience may uncritically adopt the dominant meaning of the texts and others who may be more interested in resistance simply elect not to watch or engage with the text at all.

By comparison Jonathan Gray (2008) describes fan and antifan (those people who McKinley argued elected not to engage at all) engagement of television programming for example as a form of *play*. We engage with popular culture for entertainment, for recreation, and we usually play with others. Increasingly this play takes place in online forums and blogs where people use a social network as an alibi for the creation of a community around a particular issue. Both fan and antifan discourse offer equally important insights on what we want our society to be. The way we talk about, of and through popular culture is often a discussion about society as a whole.

For Fiske (1989, 2010), popular culture can be understood as having a progressive function. Popular culture is not radical, it will not overthrow oppressive regimes but it can reflect and record the process of change. Fiske argues that meaning is not fixed and that popular culture cannot be controlled, particularly by those who seek to control it, and that 'guerilla readings are a structural necessity of the system' (p. 84). Popular culture is a site of both ideological incorporation *and* resistance.

In examining how frameworks of critical disability and disability activism have informed popular culture and vice versa, it is instructive to look at the way the evolution of disability rights has been reflected in popular culture. The progression is more cyclical than linear and often it seems to be a case of one step forwards, two steps back. Just as popular narratives introduce a character with disability with strengths and weaknesses, whose impairment is both relevant and irrelevant, another one will regurgitate the miraculous cure/triumph over adversary trope. However, disability has figured throughout popular culture and has indeed changed with the times; key moments in disability justice can be discerned, just as the shortcomings of these eras are also reflected, as will our own era's representations. Take for example, the *Star Trek* character Captain Christopher Pike. In the original 1966 series, when Pike is injured in battle, he becomes a source of revulsion to the other characters, such as his protégé Captain James Kirk who struggles to look at him. Pike's wheelchair totally encases his body, only his badly burnt face is visible.

Pike's only means of communication (via brain waves) is a large blinking light attached to the front of his wheelchair unit. However, the 2009 film remake reflects several changes related to disability and social inclusion. First, whereas the 1966 Pike was a source of pity, the 2009 character was considered a hero. Although he still relinquishes command of the ship to the able-bodied Kirk, Pike's wheelchair does not encase him and the film concludes with him 'in a low-key wheelchair, smiling, and fully functioning aside from his inability to walk' (Academic Editing Canada, 2013). It is clear that a number of social, cultural and technological changes have taken place between the *Star Trek* of 1966 and the 2009 version of the fantasy world.

Outline

While the popularity of certain texts will certainly change, the case studies throughout this book demonstrate and explore different theoretical perspectives relevant to disability studies and the disability experience. Analysis of contemporary popular culture in relation to disability adds an additional level of continuity to the book through an exploration of the impact of the specific cultural influences of the last 20 years. Throughout the book I also seek

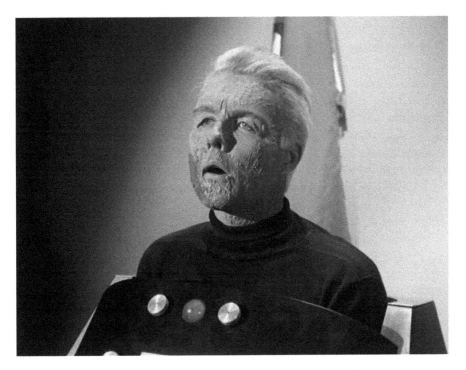

**Figure 1.1   Sean Kenney as Captain Christopher Pike in 'The Menagerie',
Star Trek 1966**

Source: © Paramount Television courtesy of Photofest.

to demonstrate the ways popular culture is cyclical and draws on conventions established in earlier popular culture artefacts.

Chapter 2, *Our Moment In Time: The Transitory and Concrete Value of Disability Toys*, uses children's toys to explore the ways popular culture both allows a variety of meanings and reflects the values of the culture that produces it. Chapter 3, *Contemporary Beauty-ism*, interrogates recent moves within critical disability studies to consider the importance of discourses of beauty, fashion and body image to people with disability. Chapter 4, *Spaces of Cultural Mediation: The Science Fiction Cinema of the Third Stage of Disability*, explores the ways science fiction cinema debates issues related to the social inclusion of people with disability in the workforce to propose a method of film analysis which takes into account the ways the social position of disability is interrogated in popular cinema.

Chapter 5, *Among the Leading Characters on Television*, applies Rosemarie Garland-Thomson's (2007) shape structures story framework to popular television to argue for an updated analysis of disability and television. Chapter 6, *Enfreaking Popular Music: Making Us Think By Making Us Feel*, considers the

13

presence of disability in popular music video discourses and reads Lady Gaga's work in particular as a disruption to the standardisation of the human form.

Chapter 7, *Controlling the Body: Sport, Disability and the Construction of Ability*, considers disability and popular sport, focusing on the Paralympics to explore social change in the context of commercialisation and likewise to argue for a recognition of the construction of ability. Chapter 8, *Disability and Spreadable Media: Access, Representation and Inspiration Porn*, explicitly considers what happens to disability culture when it encounters digitisation, focusing in particular on the criticism of so-called inspiration porn where images of people with disability are used by non-disabled people to feel better about themselves.

Throughout the book I also discuss the ways people with disability use online environments to engage in both the production and consumption cycle of popular culture to better portray their experiences and concerns. *Disability and Popular Culture* introduces readers to disability in popular culture and offers examples of popular culture to explain ideas central to the discipline of critical disability studies. While acknowledging that disability features in popular culture in ways that stigmatise, the book also aims to show the ways popular culture focuses passion, creates community and expresses defiance in the context of disability and social change. The book concludes with reflections towards this end.

Chapter 2
Our Moment In Time:
The Transitory and Concrete Value
of Disability Toys

Children's toys as popular culture objects embrace the past, present and future. Firstly, they mirror the values of the society that produce them; their shapes, colours and textures reflect what we value as important or socially acceptable at a particular moment in time. Toys also draw on a nostalgia for a culture that perhaps never existed because adults decide the culture to pass onto their children (Fleming, 1996, p. 86), and, finally, they indicate what we think the future will be like because we give toys to our children to prepare them for what we think will come. Children's toys exist in the overlap between cultural constructions of childhood innocence and the constructions that the world will eventually corrupt children. Despite children's culture being what adults want it to be, children incorporate popular culture into their play in ways that afford them agency and new ways of making meaning.

Although play is a central feature of children's culture, the high versus low culture debate rages in this arena. Children's TV must have an educational aspect to be accepted by parents and toy catalogues emphasise developmental milestones in their advertising. Henry Giroux (1998) describes children's culture as a 'sphere' where 'education, advocacy and pleasure meet to construct conceptions of what it means to be a child occupying a combination of gender, racial and class positions in society' (p. 89). While toys exist in an increasingly commercialised sphere, children's play is not necessarily commercialised (Seiter, 1995). Toy makers – especially those that offer so called transmedia or paratext toy tie-ins to television or movie conglomerates – recognise that children participate in a kind of 'audience narrativization' (Gray, 2010, p. 182) to create new opportunities and narratives around the toys.

Creativity and media literacy are important themes that run throughout this book, and they can be seen very clearly in discussions of children's toys which are often separated along distinct gender lines. As Ellen Seiter observes, children's toys are implicated in a broader cultural construction of gender:

> Children's toys and television characters copy themes of adult culture but
> present them in exaggerated versions unacceptable to adults. Gender roles

are a notorious example of this. Female characters are marked by exaggerated aesthetic codes: high pitched voices, pastel colors, frills, endless quantities of hair, and an innate capacity for sympathy. Male characters appear as superheros with enormous muscles, deep voices and an earnest and unrelenting capacity for bravery. (Seiter, 1995, pp. 10–11)

Seiter's observations play out in the bodies of two very gendered types of children's toys – Barbies and action figures such as GI Joe. However, as Seiter goes on to argue, children are creative in their play and, while they may be given mass-produced items, they use them to create popular culture, to create their own meanings and identities, not necessarily in line with consumer culture. Despite this, it is vital to teach children cultural literacy in order to contest ideological constructions.

The chapter begins with a discussion of popular culture in the form of children's toys, reflecting and validating the zeitgeist – the 'spirit of the times'. A number of toys with disability are discussed in this section, including toys used in a medical setting, transmedia offerings associated with television, movies and cartoons, Cabbage Patch-style Hal's Pals, Down Syndrome dolls and action figures. The chapter then offers case studies associated with representations of disability within the Barbie and GI Joe franchises. It argues that, whereas Barbie is accused of teaching girls about gendered existence, boys are given action figures such as GI Joe; Jason Bainbridge (2010) describes Barbie and GI Joe as occupying opposing discourses of the action figure – Barbie is the 'figure' and GI Joe the 'action' (p. 831). Whereas Barbie is immoveable, GI Joe is a 'fully articulated moveable man of action'(O'Brien, 2005, p. 5); whose body can be manipulated into real military poses.

Popular Culture Reflects the Zeitgeist

Each year toy brand American Girl release a 'girl of the year' doll, a 'character with a story about finding success in the face of challenges today' (American Girl, 2014). Promotional material for the dolls recount they ways the characters overcome challenges and learn about themselves and the world around them. In an online petition urging American Girl to release a disabled doll, Melissa Yang explains that American Girl girls of the year have introduced her to notions of diversity and asks the brand to make popular culture for and about her, a girl with disability:

> Girls of the Year come from all different places, from Hawaii to New Mexico, and they help girls learn what it's like to be someone else. Through Saige, I learned what it's like to be an artist and horseback rider. Through McKenna,

I learned what it's like to be a gymnast. Girls of the Year have helped me understand how it feels to be someone else. (Shang and Shang, 2014)

The 10-year-old with a disability describes feeling 'left out' (Zara, 2014) when it was announced that the 2014 girl of the year was Isabelle, a ballet dancer adjusting to life at a new school, and petitioned the company to produce a doll with disability to increase awareness about disability:

I don't want to be invisible or a side character that the main American Girl has to help: I want other girls to know what it's like to be me, through a disabled American Girl's story. (Shang and Shang, 2014)

Although American Girl has a number of disability accessories, including a wheelchair, hearing aid, guide dog and crutches to use with the existing dolls, Melissa Yang's petition calls for something more – recognition that disability is not an accessory and that disabled girls should have a starring role. That disability is part of diversity.

Barton and Somerville (2012) argue that children were taught race- and class-based oppression through racialised toys popular between 1880 and 1930. The absence of disabled toys between this same period, with the exception of those used in a medical setting, may have taught a different lesson in line with the exclusion of people with disability from public view characteristic of the same period. However, the idealisation of the human form is an aspect of children's toys that has been criticised for perpetuating a narrow conception of beauty, even if the absence of disability themes itself has not elicited attention.

Barton and Somerville's analysis shows that the significance of popular culture can be located temporally. Studying popular culture provides a way to understand our moment in time. Toys in particular reflect and express what an era considers important and offer valuable insights by documenting cultural eras. The availability of multicultural Barbies and GI Joes illustrates this point. While both toys were initially launched as white, changing ideas of multiculturalism are reflected in the increasing diversity of these toys. However, initial toys were little more than white toys in disguise, being modelled on the original form but dipped in dark paint. Barbie's 1967 offensively named friend 'Coloured Francie' was the same as white Barbies, simply dyed black or brown. This was not unique to Barbie; according to Karen Hall, the 1960s black/brown GI Joe unintentionally created a system of white supremacy because they looked identical to the first – white – GI Joe. However, things were beginning to change, and, in 1970, an African American head sculpt was introduced to the GI Joe range (Hall, 2004, p. 37). Mattell continued to introduce Black and Hispanic Barbies throughout the 1980s, and eventually hired multicultural consultants in the 1990s when they introduced their Shani line. The consultants recommended slight bodily differences between black and white Barbies.

Reflecting on Coloured Francie, Ann Du Cille (1994) is unable to answer the question whether a black Barbie that looks the same as a white one is better than no black Barbie at all. She describes the first black Barbie she saw as 'the most beautiful thing I had ever seen' – an 'Other' like herself (p. 64). These issues can similarly be applied to toys with disabilities.

In 1995 *The Advertising Age* described the focus on 'diversity toy marketing' in Toys "R" Us catalogues as reflective of changing social demographics and attitudes (Multicultural Toys For Children of the '90s, 1995). Although explicitly referring to race, the allusion towards culture could refer to the emergence of disability-themed toys. Toys "R" Us catalogues now include a section for 'differently able kids' which features both toys made for a mass market that are particularly suited to children with disability and those specifically modified for children with disabilities (see Toys "R" Us, 2014). The presence of this section again reflects a change in social attitudes. When institutional care was considered the only option for children with disabilities, they were often not given toys to play with. However, as people began refusing to put their children into institutions during the 1970s, opting to care for them at home, the importance of toys and play for children with disabilities began to be recognised (see Noah's Ark, 2013).

Jack Nachbar and Kevin Lause argue that popular culture reflects the values of the culture in which it was produced and make a distinction between the transitory and concrete values that appear within popular culture:

> The study of popular culture as a reflective mirror of its audience must focus upon two aspects of this zeitgeist – the "transitory" and the "concrete". The zeitgeist which characterizes a particular era is composed of "transitory" attitudes and perspectives which last only as long as the era itself and then fade from view – perhaps to return in later times, perhaps not. But an era's zeitgeist also expresses deep-seated, highly significant "concrete" beliefs and values which transcend the specific time period and represent the fundamental character of the culture itself. Most elements of popular culture reflect both of these zeitgeist levels in important ways. (Nachbar and Lause, 1992, p. 5)

The toys under discussion in this chapter reflect both transitory and concrete cultural values and hold a mirror to the concerns of the eras which produced them – they also offer us an insight into more long-standing cultural beliefs about masculinity and femininity. GI Joe's 'Mike Power Atomic Man' reflects transitory attitudes related to the Vietnam War and the reintegration of disabled vets to society, while Barbie's 'Share a Smile Becky' transitory values can be closely tied to the introduction of disability discrimination legislation. However, both toys retain concrete values regarding masculinity and femininity in particular, with related consequences for the cultural construction of disability.

A Selected History of Disability Toys

Despite key studies into the importance of toys in everyday life, the construction of childhood and the perpetuation of gender roles, there is a distinct lack of research into disability toys from a cultural studies perspective. Indeed, when it comes to disability and toys, the majority of academic discussion centres on developmental psychology, physiotherapy and the construction of special toys for children with 'special needs'. In short the discussion is entirely medicalised.

Jeffrey Goldstein's (2005) edited collection *Toys, Games, and Media* explores the changing nature of toys, games and media across time and place, focusing on issues such as the effect digital media has on imaginative play and the commercial exploitation of children. The book includes a chapter on toys and disability which interrogates the question as to whether toys should be adapted for children with disabilities or if these children should adapt to the commercially available toys (Fabregat, Costa, and M. Romero, 2005). While the chapter introduces a welcome consideration of disability in terms of diversity, it does not explore the changing nature of disability toys across time. As Sharon Snyder and David Mitchell argue in *Cultural Locations of Disability* (2006), the culturally pervasive nature of disability has been 'filtered through the perspectives … of those who locate disability on the outermost margins of human value' (p. 21). Snyder and Mitchell demonstrate the way cultural understandings of disability are influenced by institutions and practices from charity to film, institutionalised care and medical research in ways that medicalise disability as biologically deviant. We can see this filtering occurring in children's popular culture.

Disability toys and comics are often used in an awareness raising capacity or are applauded for their inspirational qualities. Comics as a form of popular media have long displayed a heightened fascination with disability – from superheroes and villains to secret identities, to Superman fighting against polio to Wonder Woman explaining how an iron lung works. Yet the earliest disability toys of the twentieth century are arguably icons of medical culture rather than popular culture. Toys have been used throughout history to explain surgical procedures and other interventions to children such as soft toys with cochlear implants in the 1990s and toy dogs fitted with sitting sockets in the 1960s. In another example, dolls and teddy bears with callipers were used in hospitals to teach children about polio between the 1930s and '50s, as this entry from the British Science Museum explains:

> Being in hospital was frightening, and many children found it difficult to understand what was happening to their bodies. What could you do to explain

their conditions, and to reassure both children and their worried parents that the treatments could help them? Staff at the hospital used … everyday-looking toys to prepare and encourage children and their families. The dolls helped to personalise the process. They were dressed in hospital clothes, some accompanied by their teddy bears, and in beds made with hospital sheets and blankets. One was even cocooned in a tiny iron lung. These mini-patients were an attempt to create reassurance in the face of quite drastic and sometimes painful treatments. (Ceramic teaching doll to show treatment for polio, England, 1930–1950)

Similarly, entries for toys, dolls, comics and teddy bears on *The Museum of Disability History*, *Digital-Disability.com* and *Everybody: An Artefact History of Disability in America* reveal that toys have been used throughout history to communicate cultural ideas regarding disability, dependency and culture. With the exception of medicalised doctors' and nurses' kits which began to be featured during the 1940s, a content analysis of Billy and Ruth toy catalogues between 1930 and 1963 reveal an absence of disability-themed toys until a Three Blind Mice Talking Toy in 1955. The next to appear is the culturally significant Mr Magoo Toy Car in 1961 (see catalogues archived on Mueller, n.d).

Quincy Magoo, affectionately called Mr Magoo, has been the target of several disability protests. The short statured cartoon character, created in 1949, constantly finds himself in comical situations due to his refusal to accept that he is near blind. He is also an example of transmedia popular culture. Initially a theatrical short throughout the 1950s, Mr Magoo was repurposed for television in the 1960s and remade as a movie in 1997 (see Pierce, 1997 for a discussion of the protest surrounding Mr Magoo). In 1962 the children's toy of Mr Magoo driving a car was met with protest from people who were blind and vision impaired for stereotyping their impairment (Mr Magoo Toy Car, 1960s). The 1997 movie bombed at the box office following disability protests.

Indeed, the earliest mobilisations of disability rights groups highlighted the importance of children's toys and their associated transmedia to the ideological construction of disability. As the toy industry has become increasingly commercialised, disability toys have begun emerging more often through transmedia cross overs with television shows and movies such as the Laurel and Hardy electronic drawing set (1962) the Ironside game and van and the Dr Who Dalek figurine. Dan Flemming identifies the ways children use transmedia toys to create their own narratives using *Star Wars* toys. He finds that the toys, while replicas of the characters in the *Star Wars* films, allow children to expand the story world in ways relevant to themselves:

A child looking at a crazily diverse collection of small toy figures from the Star Wars universe in the late 1970s was being offered a set of questions about the white male hero's relationships with furry dwarfs, hairy giants, intelligent machines and a human community of various colours and creeds. Unlike what happens in traditional fairy tales, those others do not constitute a supporting menagerie compliant to the hero's will but rather a complex imaginary "culture" to which the hero has to accommodate in order to achieve anything. (Fleming, 1996, p. 100)

While toys with disabilities may have functioned as peripheral characters in the *Star Wars* narrative world, in children's play they can become the leading characters (see Gray, 2010). Children therefore become prosumers, a hybrid mix of producer/consumer in the use of toys as avatars to play out their identities and relationships with self and others. In *Convergence Culture*, Henry Jenkins observes that transmedia storytelling utilises the strengths of a number of mediums (for example comics, films, television, games, toys) whereby any product is a point of entry for a different audience. He argues that reading across all media sustains a new depth of experience and more comprehensive story information.

One example is the *Six Million Dollar Man* which has a transmedia narrative stretching from the 1972 novel *Cyborg* on which the story was based through to the 1970s telemovie, television series, spin-off series (*Bionic Woman*) and action figure. More recently, a comic book was launched in 2011. An official *Six Million Dollar Man* action figure was distributed by Kenner Toys in 1975, the same year that real life amputee and private investigator, hostage negotiator and 'trouble consultant' Jay J. Armes released his autobiography *J.J. Armes, Investigator: The World's Most Successful Private Eye*. Armes, who lost his hands in a railroad accident as a youth, provided a real life embodiment of the *Six Million Dollar Man*.

In 1976, Ideal Toys modelled an entire line of action figures on Armes. Indeed, J. Jay Armes embodies the same hyper-masculinity and resourcefulness of other action figures popular at the time and since. He is as strong as He-Man, has as many attachments and disguises as Action Man and was as patriotic as GI Joe. These action figures are broadly defined by physical attributes associated with strength and overcoming enemies. J. Jay Armes is the ultimate action figure, always ready for action because his body is effectively the action. His gun and hook accessories attach directly to his body making *him* the ultimate weapon. If children's toys exaggerate and hyperbolise adult culture in ways unacceptable to adults, then J. Jay Armes is an exaggeration of rehabilitation post-disablement and the association between masculinity and action. J. Jay Armes is the hyperbolisation of the action figure itself. While Bignell (2000) describes Action Man (the UK version of GI Joe) as the 'title of a coherent mythical world' (p. 231), J. Jay Armes takes this world to a new level.

Like the *Six Million Dollar Man* and his real life name sake, the Jay J. Armes toy was resourceful:

No matter what the situation or crisis required, a kid could modify his Jay J. Armes doll with: 2 suction cups for climbing walls; a wrist-locked magnet for hanging onto steel structures; an implanted machete to cut his way out of tough situations; a pair of false hands for undercover roles, so as to look undistinguished from the rest of the crowd; a prosthesis that converts to a pistol; and a pair of spring loaded hooks. (Miller, n.d.)

Of course these accessories represent more money going to the toy makers. However, it was unlikely families could afford to buy the entire range. As a result many children would merge transmedias to play with toys across specific brands to create new narratives (Bainbridge, 2010, p. 385). Despite the fact that action figures are essentially dolls, the imaginative play they elicit is based outside in unfamiliar territories (Bignell, 2000). Girls' dolls, by comparison, have as many accessories, vehicles and play sets but these are usually located within domestic spheres.

Dolls[1]

While dolls have historically been made to replicate the human form, they are generally conceived as white and able-bodied. Doris Wilkinson (1987) explains that 'the word doll is derived from the Greek eiddon meaning idol' (p. 20) and outlines the ways dolls reflect changing cultural beliefs about femininity, class and religion. Dolls are not inconsequential; they occupy an important cultural position in the dissemination and reinforcement of normative values regarding race, class and gender and, I would argue, disability.

During the 1980s Mattel introduced a multiracial series of Cabbage Patch-style 19-inch dolls called Hal's Pals that had a variety of disabilities:

In addition to Hal, who doesn't have a left leg and is the only doll who has been named, there is a ballerina wearing hearing aids, a boy in a gray warm-up suit in a wheelchair, and a girl with leg braces and canes. The fifth disabled Pal, a girl, is visually impaired and comes with a red-tipped cane and guide dog. The two other dolls, a preppy boy and a Madonna look-alike, do not appear disabled. However, they can be bought with the various accessories, such as the wheelchair. (Inquirer Wire Services, 1986)

---

1   Some material in this section has appeared in print before at Ellis, K. (2012). Complicating a Rudimentary List of Characteristics: Communicating Disability with Down Syndrome Dolls. *Media Culture Journal* 15(5), http://journal.media-culture.org. au/index.php/mcjournal/article/viewArticle/544.

At the time Paul Valentine, a toy-industry analyst, claimed the dolls would not have longevity because they were unlikely to be embraced by children who tended to be 'cruel':

> Handicapped children already feel different. I doubt that they would want to feel even more different, to have a doll specially geared to them that is not part of the mass culture. (Valentine cited on Timberlake, 1986)

While Valentine's critique fails to grasp the importance of disability representation across all aspects of popular culture, he does recognise the ways people turn mass culture into popular culture through meaning making and identity formation. As Fiske (1989) notes, a problematic relationship exists between the commercial and the popular. While popular culture is criticised for its commercialisation and for perpetuating damaging dominant ideologies, people use commodities to construct meanings of the self and social identity and relationships.

Down Syndrome dolls, which became available in the early 2000s, bridge the medical and cultural approaches to disability toys. These dolls, based on composites of a number of children with Down Syndrome, are in stark contrast to dolls popularly available which assume a normative representation and embrace bodily perfection. Helga Parks, CEO of HEST, describes the dolls as a realistic representation of nine physical features of Down Syndrome. Likewise, Donna Moore of Downi Creations employed a designer to oversee the production of the dolls which represent 13 features of Down Syndrome (Velasquez, 2007). Achieving the physical features of Down Syndrome is significant because Parks and Moore wanted children with the condition to recognise themselves:

> When a child with Down's syndrome (sic) picks up a regular doll, he doesn't see himself, he sees the world's perception of "perfect". Our society is so focused on bodily perfection. (Cresswell, 2008)

Despite these motivations, studies show that children with Down Syndrome prefer to play with 'typical dolls' that do not reflect the physical characteristics of Down Syndrome (Cafferty, 2012, p. 49). According to Cafferty, it is possible that children prefer typical dolls because they are 'more attractive' (p. 49). Similar studies of diverse groups of children have shown that children prefer to play with dolls they perceive as fitting into social concepts of beauty (Abbasi, 2012). These deeply embedded cultural notions of beauty – which exclude disability – are communicated from childhood (Blair and Shalmon 15).

Many bodies, not just those deemed disabled, do not conform to these cultural standards. Cultural ideals of beauty and an idealisation of the human body according to increasingly narrow parameters are becoming conflated with

DISABILITY AND POPULAR CULTURE

conceptions of normality (Wendell, 1996, p. 86). Recognition of disability as subject to cultural rejection allows us to see 'beauty and normalcy [as] a series of practices and positions [taken] in order to avoid the stigmatisation of ugliness and abnormality' (Garland-Thomson, 2001). The exaggerated features of Down Syndrome or Downi Creation dolls problematise the expectation that people with disability strive to appear as non-disabled as possible and, in turn, highlights that some people, such as those with Down Syndrome, cannot 'pass' as non-disabled and must therefore navigate a life and community that is not welcoming. Yet the dolls themselves have been heavily criticised by some sectors of the community:

> Apparently some people upon coming across [Down Syndrome dolls] were offended. […] Still, it's curious, and telling, what gives offense. Was it the shock of seeing a doll not modeled on the normative form that caused such offense? Or the assumption that any representation of Down Syndrome must naturally intend ridicule? Either way, it would seem that we might benefit from an examination of such reactions – especially as they relate to instances of the idealisation of the human form that dolls […] represent. (Faulkner, 2008)

When Loraine Faulkner describes public criticism of dolls designed to look like they have Down Syndrome, she draws attention to the need for an examination of the way discourses of disability are communicated. The dolls are also an example of unpopular culture, with Downi Creations shutting doors and Down Syndrome dolls experiencing a cruel and malicious backlash.

However, the dolls have been rebranded as 'scientific' dolls and sold on Amazon. While Downi Creations has discontinued their doll and Helga Parks (whose website www.downsyndromedolls.com is still operational) told me in an email that she has experienced an extended backlash against the dolls, a new manufacturer emerged in 2013. Initially called Dolls for Downs and now renamed Extra Special Dolls, the company seeks to de-medicalise Down Syndrome dolls and perhaps return to the focus on beauty in dolls. According to their website:

> Our exquisite doll faces reflect the lovely features found in individuals with Down Syndrome. From the sparkling, almond shaped eyes, gently curved noses and down turned lips to the smaller, lower set ears and generally flattened forehead, we believe that we have captured the essence and playful personality of a child up for anything! (ESD, 2014)

Children's toys as popular culture artefacts reflect the values of the society that produce them. While it may be too early to tell whether these new dolls created in 2013 will have longevity, the unpopularity of Downi Creations and

HEST's Down Syndrome dolls reveal something about the culture in which they were produced.

Barbie

Boasting a cult following of adults and children alike, images of Barbie appear frequently in popular culture across television, advertising, the internet, cinema, music and art. From internet sites and Facebook fan pages about the doll to sites about actual women engaging plastic surgery to look more like the doll (see www.cindyjackson.com) to the 1974 decision to rename part of Times Square Barbie Boulevard for a week – Barbie's cultural significance is clear. However, Barbie is a 'site of unresolved tension' between progressive and regressive images of women in popular, children's and consumer culture (Fleming, 1996, p. 42).

Barbie is not a fixed cultural text, her image, body shape and colour have changed in response to social and political changes. Although Barbie has come to be synonymous with blonde hair, the first Barbie was available as either a blonde or a brunette (1959) and wore a black and white striped swimming costume. Her hair was in a ponytail. In 1971 her eyes were adjusted to look forwards rather than to the side, and while her waist was reduced during the 1980s, it was again increased to 'more realistic proportions' during the 1990s to compensate for changes in fashion. Her teeth and smile have changed over the years and she has gained a belly button.

While these changes are largely superficial and located within her physical body, Barbie has also been influenced by key historical moments and movements. Although Mary Rogers (1999) explains these have little to do with a social justice ethos on the side of the manufacturer. Drawing on Seiter's (1995) argument that children creatively consume mass culture to play with shifting identity, multicultural and feminist themes can be read into Barbie's shifting diversity. For Rogers (1999), Barbie 'exemplifies contradictions enough to appeal to a wide range of consumers' (p. 89). There have been a number of culturally diverse Barbies varying in skin colour, such as Coloured Francie (1967–8), Christie (1968–2005), and Shani, Nasha and Nichelle (1992–1999). As previously discussed, Francie was criticised for being made with the same head mould as a white Barbie, so Christie, who was released the following year, is considered the first true African American Barbie.

Accessories have also changed in response to social and political changes. A book entitled *How to Lose Weight* was included with two outfits during the 1960s, and contained advice such as 'don't eat'. It came with toy scales permanently set to 110 pounds. With regards to her employment prospects, Barbie is famous for having 130 careers, stretching back into the 1960s when she was released as a surgeon.

However, Barbie remains a contested image in feminist cultural analysis, being described as 'a symbol of women's oppression under capitalism and patriarchy' (Toffoletti, 2007, p. 62). Barbie's unnaturally lean and busty figure has been blamed for unrealistic body image and anorexia among young girls and the increased incidence of breast implants. A 1977 article takes a disparaging stance, predicting that Barbie could produce a generation of girls that resist getting married, having children and indeed responsibility of any kind (Cox, 1977). Further, critics argue that Barbie turns girls into consumers by teaching them that in order to succeed they must look good:

> Barbie signifies fixed gender roles, heterosexual norms and consumerist values to which women must strive. Barbie is said to teach girls the codes of femininity through standards of dress, bodily ideas and modes of behaviour. She is rigid and slender, always smiling and immaculately groomed and attired, mostly in pink. (Toffoletti, 2007, p. 60)

Barbie's 'friend', 'Share a Smile Becky', uses a wheelchair and challenges these fixed roles, norms and meanings. Mattel first introduced Share a Smile Becky in 1996 at the Very Special Arts Gallery in Washington, DC. Together with Toys "R" Us, the toy manufacturer donated $10,000 to disability charities. With more than 150 children with disabilities in attendance, the doll was reportedly 'welcomed by national disability rights leaders' at the time (Mattel, 1997). However, other people with disability responded less favourably:

> "The name makes me want to gag", said Leslie Heller, who has cerebral palsy. Nadina LaSpina, who had polio, said, "It shows they can make money off of us". "We'll see where it's marketed", said Deborah Yanagisawa, who is blind. "It will be in the hospital gift shops". (Martin, 1997)

In an editorial for *The New York Times*, Douglas Martin described such negative reactions from the disability community as evidence of a 'a new militant attitude among many of the disabled' who were using popular culture to advocate for a better quality of life and better public understanding of disability as a condition rather than illness (Martin, 1997). Mattell themselves described the doll in a series of press releases:

> Barbie® doll's hip and very cool disabled friend who is a photographer for her high school yearbook. She comes with a pretend camera so she can take "pictures" at all school events. Becky doll uses a red and silver realistically designed wheelchair and keeps in style wearing a trendy fashion ensemble accessorized

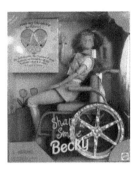

Figure 2.1 Share A Smile Becky

Source: BECKY and associated trademarks and trade dress are owned by, and used under permission from, Mattel. © Mattel. All Rights Reserved.

with red stud earrings, red framed sunglasses, and a brown backpack that hangs on the back of her wheelchair.

Becky also appears in a new book entitled, Barbie, The New Counselor, published by Golden Books, where she works as a camp counselor with Barbie. This emphasizes the Becky doll's leadership abilities and sends a powerful message to kids. In addition, Becky will appear in the Detective Barbie CD-ROM where she helps the Barbie doll solve mysteries using her incredible computer skills to uncover clues. (tmeronek, 2010)

When Share a Smile Becky was released, the doll received vast media coverage from outlets such as CNN, USA Today and the Washington Post. In *Barbie Culture*, Mary Rogers argues that keeping Barbie in the news is a form of 'virtual advertising' adopted by Mattel in order to infiltrate consumer consciousness. She describes Mattel's introduction of Share a Smile Becky and the associated coverage of disability issues – both positive and negative – as its most successful example of this strategy (Rogers, 1999, p. 99). Jamie Berke (2011) describes the doll as the event which most 'excited the disability community in 1997'. Indeed, the doll sold out in two weeks, forcing Mattell to go back into production (Mattel, 1997).

Becky has been interpreted in a number of different ways. For example, whereas an article in *USA Today* criticised her for her wardrobe, cleavage and beauty (Shiparo 1997 cited in Rogers, 1999), adult bloggers reflect on the importance of Becky to their sense of selves growing up and coming to terms with their disability (Disability Horizons, 2013). Rosemarie Garland-Thomson holds Becky up as an ironic example of the ways women with disability are banished from feminine ideals in ways that are both beneficial and limiting:

The disabled Becky is dressed and poised for agency, action, and creative engagement with the world. In contrast, the prototypical Barbie performs excessive femininity in her restrictive gowns, crowns and push up bras. So while Becky implies on the one hand that disabled girls are purged from the feminine economy, on the other hand she also suggests that disabled girls might be liberated from those oppressive and debilitating scripts. (Garland-Thomson, 2011, p. 32)

She argues that while Becky may be empowered because she is not subject to the disabling impact of women's fashion and clothing restrictions, a broader social cost may be that she 'loses her sense of identity as a feminine sexual being' (p. 32). Thus Becky and Barbie open a site for interrogation of gender roles within the context of disability embodiment.

With her purple wheelchair and pink leggings, Becky epitomised '90s street fashion, while Barbie's 'unpractical clothes' have been provided as evidence of her continued subordination of women. For Garland-Thomson (2004), Becky's comfortable clothes signal towards a feminist critique of Barbie as the fashion icon as Becky casts off the hyperbole of feminine fashion with all its restrictions for clothes that allow movement and agency (Garland-Thomson, 2004, p. 89).

Although Barbie identifies as able-bodied, if her proportions were extended to the life size equivalent she would be classified as disabled – she would be unable to stand upright and, like the doll, would topple forwards due to her pointy feet. Ironically, Becky's packaging features Becky sitting between Barbie and Christie who are both standing. While in reality Barbie and Christie would be unable to stand, Becky is secure and independently upright in her chair. Humorously, a warning on the back of the packaging reads: 'Barbie and Christie dolls cannot stand alone.' Becky has flat feet and is one of the few Barbies whose legs bend at the knees (Garland-Thompson 2004, p. 89). Therefore, unlike the 'multicultural' Barbies such as Francie – who are arguably nothing more than white Barbies dipped in black or brown dye (du Cille, 1994, p. 52) – Becky is a different physical construction and, as a result, is more stable than non-disabled Barbie.

However, Becky's wheelchair could not fit into a number of Barbie's accessories, including most notably the Barbie Dream House. This article from the *Seattle Times* reveals the way accessibility became an important issue through the body of Share a Smile Becky, admittedly an issue Mattell was able to leverage to stay in the public's attention.

Amid much ballyhoo and a drum roll of press releases last month, perky "Share a Smile Becky", as toymaker Mattel has dubbed her, made her debut as the newest member of the Barbie doll family. Advocates for people with disabilities heralded Becky's arrival, because youngsters who use wheelchairs now would have a doll just like them. The doll is intended to change attitudes about people with disabilities, Mattel said proudly. But, alas, Barbie and friends have not read the 1990 Americans with Disabilities Act, which requires accessible entrances for wheelchairs. Becky's wheelchair, it turns out, doesn't fit through the doors of the Barbie dollhouse. (Gilje, 1997)

Becky's exclusion from the Barbie Dream House and other accessories was an important feature in raising awareness around the politicisation of disability in wider society and highlights Becky's emergence from a culture that was in the process of becoming more inclusive. Following the introduction of Disability Discrimination Acts internationally during the 1990s, many buildings had to be retrofitted with lifts. Even now, a quarter century later, a large number of buildings remain inaccessible. Becky, like Coloured Francie, was the product of the social conditions in which she was produced.

Action Figures

Karen O'Brien (2005), author of *Warman's G.I. Joe Field Guide: Values and Identification*, argues that 'GI Joe accomplished for boys in 1964 what Barbie accomplished five years earlier for girls – it allowed boys to role-play any situation their imaginations dreamed up' (p. 5). Like Barbie, GI Joe has adapted to historical, social, cultural and even economic changes. In 1964 he was released as an open-ended military concept possessing a 12 inch body, battle scar below his right eye, athletic figure and a backwards thumbnail. However, as military readiness began losing cultural currency, GI Joe, who had previously enjoyed a massive popularity, plummeted in sales. He was rebranded as a civilian man of action in 1969, given flocked hair and beard in 1970, a 'kung fu' grip in 1974, and briefly as part-man-part-machine Mike Power Atomic Man. When plastics became more expensive as a result of the Opec Oil crisis, he was released as an 8-inch figure in 1977 and, in order to compete with *Star Wars* figurines, he was further reduced to 3¾ inches in the late 1970s.

Karen Hall's analysis of the body of GI Joe reflects many of the concerns of disability studies. She cites David Harvey's assertion that the body is both an unfinished project and a relational 'thing' that gathers its meanings from outside forces to consider the shifting notions of masculinity. This is communicated through the changing shape of GI Joe who, despite a number of changes in height, skin colour, hair, 'kung fu' grip and ability, remains firmly embedded in the cultural zeitgeist as an icon of masculinity. Although Hall does not mention Mike Power, her argument that the body of GI Joe gains its meaning from outside social and historical forces applies to a disability reading of this member of the GI Joe Adventure Team.

As the first socially accepted boy's doll, GI Joe initiated an entirely new category of boy's toys that would be embraced by toy makers and movie franchises. Significantly, both Barbie's and GI Joe's success rests in their accessories and associated characters. Both embrace a marketing strategy described by the razor/razor blade metaphor where the doll represents the originally bought razor and the multitude of accessories are the metaphorical razor blades needed to operate the initial purchase. GI Joe's first release represented the four branches of the US armed forces – army, navy, marine and air force. GI Joe has both adapted to contemporary forms of military readiness throughout its history and offers a 'virtual map of the cultural zeitgeist' (Bainbridge, 2010, p. 382). Just as Barbie has been accused of instilling negative body images in young girls, academic studies have hypothesised the long term impact of exposure to hyper masculinised dolls such as GI Joe on male body image (see Diedrichs and Lee, 2010). GI Joe's masculinity is inscribed in his muscular body and trademark battle scar:

> The masculine ideal that GI Joe was engineered to adhere to is ready for action at the expense of having access to the full range of physical and emotional experience. His battle scar is evidence of an earlier meeting with the enemy, which taught him to control his fear, and his stoic expression is masculinity's behavioral outcome. (Hall, 2004, p. 50)

While the wound was intended as a way to trademark the body of the doll against forgeries, the scar has taken on very 'manly' connotations. Battle wounds work to increase an audience perception of masculinity and allow us to gaze upon the male body in a non-erotic way. Mike Power retained his battle scar as homage to his military roots; however, it was moved to the left side of his face. Indeed Mike Power's atomic limbs necessitated a new body sculpt.

While the first GI Joe capitalised on a cultural sense of masculinised military readiness and stood for isolated individualism, eventually this feature would plague the toy as parents adopted an anti-war sentiment and protested against the Vietnam War directly to the Toy Fare of 1966 (Walsh, 2005, p. 199). As a result, GI Joe became a *re*action figure, rebranding as an adventurer in 1969. This reaction would follow GI Joe throughout the rest of his career as a number of other action figures adversely affected sales of the action figure associated with the military. GI Joe's shift from an armed forces character to a civilian adventurer has been described as his 'castration' (see Hall, 2004 for a full discussion).

The little known story in this discussion is the role disability played in the GI Joe franchise. Mike Power the Atomic Man was actually the first GI Joe to be given a name. In an attempt to diversify its image and attract customers away from other action figures emerging at the time that were not associated with a pro war sentiment, this iteration of the action figure capitalised on the *Six Million Dollar Man* movie and television show by remaking GI Joe as a superhuman disabled member of an adventure team.

Mike Power's right eye, arm and left leg were prosthetic or, as Hasbro termed, 'atomic' (they could not use the term bionic due to copyright restrictions). The toy's eye flashed reflective material in the top of its head and his arm could propel a hand held helicopter attachment. When Mike Power ran he used only his atomic leg. While Mike Power could only be described as superhuman, disability featured importantly in his backstory:

> Mike Power was born with disabled limbs. He refused to accept them and spent his life developing atomic parts for his body. His atomic leg allowed him to run 200 miles per hour, his atomic arm could lift 10,000 pounds and his atomic eye could see through six feet of solid steel. He decided to join the Adventure Team and demonstrated his abilities, convincing G.I. Joe he had what was needed. Later he and G.I. Joe encountered and recruited Bulletman to the team. (GI Joe meets the Amazing Atomic Man!)

Tobin Siebers's (2008) discussion of the problem of the cyborg provides opportunity to reflect on the rhetoric of this character blurb. As Siebers explains, despite the initial need for a prosthesis, cyborgs who are constructed as more than human in popular culture are 'not disabled'(p. 63). Mike Power is a cyborg in the vein of the *Six Million Dollar Man* and possesses extraordinary abilities. When GI Joe first meets Mike Power in a 1975 advertisement "GI Joe meets the Amazing Atomic Man!", he is unimpressed by Power's quiet and reserved nature, doubting he has what it takes to be part of the team. Power 'removes his suit to reveal his atomic eye, atomic arm and atomic leg' (GI Joe meets the Amazing Atomic Man!) and when GI Joe puts him to the test his amazing abilities become apparent. The advertisement concludes with Mike Power high-fiving the rest of the Adventure Team. From then on Power wears short pants and short sleeve shirts to expose his bionic limbs that were modelled in clear plastic and given internal workings (Wheeler, n.d.). By comparison, *Six Million Dollar Man* Steve Austin's prosthetic body is indistinguishable from the biological human form and covered with clothing.

Mike Power is not just a technological marvel; he is shown in the comic advertisement sitting in a wheelchair creating the technology that would eventually become his atomic limbs. Power has a further edge on Steve Austin in that he developed the technology to make him superhuman himself, while Austin was delivered by and therefore always indebted to the government agency OSI (Office of Scientific Intelligence). In this way Power, like J. Jay Armes discussed earlier in the chapter, has more agency exhibiting resourcefulness in the creation of their own fate.

Perhaps we can think of Mike Power as little more than what disability theorists have derided as supercripples or characters with disability who achieve social integration through hard work, determination and overcoming their 'inferior bodies'. The character blurb cited earlier certainly embraces that rhetoric, a concept that would also appeal to the parents buying the toy for their children.

GI Joe appeared at a significant juncture of American social beliefs around masculinity. While the original toy embraced Second World War-masculinity, the adventure team, led by Mike Power, displayed a shifting masculinity characterised by an individualistic resourcefulness. The change in social milieu brought about by the Vietnam War had a significant impact on public reception of the action figure, just as it did on disability politics. Hall (2004) describes the mood shifting to 'focus on the individual, as if the crisis of the historical moment was defined by crisis on the individual level rather than the national or ideological' (p. 37). As a result, sales of the military ready toy plummeted.

At the same time, returning Vietnam veterans are recognised as having a significant impact on the disability civil rights movement in America. The 1973 Rehabilitation Act which established government support for rehabilitation and recreational programs for people with disability is described by Kim Neilsen was being driven by 'the needs of Vietnam veterans' (Neilsen, 2012, p. 166). Dan Goodley (2011) locates the emergence of a minority model of disability within the social milieu of Black civil rights, queer politics and returning Vietnam vets. The minority model seeks to challenge ableism or the 'social biases against people whose bodies function differently from those bodies considered to be "normal"' (p. 12).

Martin Norden (1994) sees this social context being reflected in films of the era which represented disability. While he sees a rehabilitative focus arising, he argues that the majority of films continue to isolate disability as abnormal. As the use of technology rose during the 1970s and 1980s, cultural images of disability began reflecting an interest in the 'techno marvel' disabled character (Norden, 1994, p. 293). These characters, on television (the *Six Million Dollar Man*, the *Bionic Woman*) and movies (*Star Wars*, *Robocop*), reframe prosthesis as both superhuman and less than human. These characters' capabilities are enhanced beyond normal human limits using various artificial body parts. Arthur Asa Berger (1980) describes the pleasure in watching *The Six Million Dollar Man* as located in the realisation that Steve Austin has escaped death, and so we might too (p. 116). He sees the narrative displaying an uncertainty about technology but notes that, whereas Frankenstein as a similar cultural figure represents death brought to life, Austin is life kept from death. Mike Power takes this pleasure a step further because he engineered this escape from death himself.

Although over 1 million units of Mike Power were sold in the first year of release (Robonut, n.d.), the action figure was short-lived as GI Joe went on to react to other cultural trends. Together with GI Joe, Mike Power recruited Bulletman to the Adventure Team a move which competed with superheroes becoming popular at the time.

Conclusion

In his 2009 documentary television series *James' May Toy Stories*, James May described the story of toys as 'the story of everything'. He suggested that if future archaeologists wanted to find out what life was like in the twentieth century they need only look into a toy box (cited in Bainbridge, 2010, p. 829). Indeed, popular culture is linked to the zeitgeist. Toys as popular culture are not inconsequential, they offer us a way to understand the values of the culture that produced them. They also offer insight into what a culture thinks the future will be like because we give them to children.

The popular culture of disability toys began as a history of medical culture. While toys, dolls and teddy bears have been used in medical settings to illustrate surgical procedures or the attachment of particular prosthetics, gradually, throughout the twentieth century, specific disability toys began emerging in mass culture. These were turned into popular culture through the imaginative and creative play of children. Some such as Hal's Pals and Down Syndrome Dolls were created specifically for children with disabilities, others – notably the J. Jay Armes and Mike Power Atomic Man action figures and Share a Smile Becky – were intended for the wider market.

As Nachbar and Lause argue, popular culture is made up of two distinct values – the transitory and the concrete. Transitory values can be directly tied to a particular era, while concrete values are more permanent and transcend the time period in which they were made. As I discussed throughout this chapter, Share a Smile Becky reflects the transitory moment of the introduction of disability legislation in several Western nations throughout the 1990s while also communicating more concrete values about feminine beauty. Similarly, disabled action figures such as GI Joe's Mike Power Atomic Man and Ideal Toy's Jay J. Armes communicate concrete values that associate masculinity with strength and resourcefulness while delving into transitory values regarding injured veterans seeking a place within mainstream society. It is intriguing that Share a Smile Becky has gained so much attention in disability, feminist and blogging circles, even almost 20 years after its release but that Atomic Man is largely unremarked despite its key position in reorienting the GI Joe brand to a more acceptable cultural image. If the toys we give our children reflect the best aspects of our past and communicate what we think the future will be like, both point towards a greater social inclusion of people with disabilities in education and employment.

Chapter 3
Contemporary Beauty-ism

When Abercrombie and Fitch were criticised in the media for firing Riam Dean, an employee with disability, for violating their 'look policy', their Chief Executive Mike Jeffries unapologetically described the fashion giant's approach to attracting the 18–22 year old market, '… we go for the cool kids. A lot of people don't belong and can't belong. Are we exclusionary? Absolutely' (Jeffries cited in Hoyle, 2009). A pursuit of physical perfection is evident in their advertising materials, topless male shop-front models, and scantily-dressed shop assistants. Their exclusionary ethos was further highlighted by their discriminatory firing of Dean who had offered to wear a cardigan to obscure her prosthetic arm. She went on to win a case of discrimination against them. Abercrombie and Fitch thus set a benchmark in the use of the beauty myth against which others in the industry are compared. In the process, they became a target of media critique. For example, Diesel, another significant figure in fashion, has recently been described as 'not Abercrombie and Fitch' following its focus on diversity in recent campaigns.

The increasing conflation of the 'ideal' with the 'norm' evident in fashion imagery and popular culture offers an opportunity to reassess the social and cultural construction of disability as being outside parameters of beauty and perfection. Naomi Wolf identifies the existence of a 'beauty myth' in media and popular culture which can be equated to youthful, slender and flawless bodies in her seminal third wave feminist book *The Beauty Myth*. Further, Wolf argues that this myth was invented by a male power structure to prevent women from achieving the feminist ideals of the 1970s. By viewing disability as an example of being outside the beauty myth in this context, disability becomes an experience that non-disabled people can relate to on the basis of their own experiences of social discrimination regarding beauty, or the pressures they feel to be youthful, slender and flawless (see Garland-Thomson, 1995). However, the notion that people with disability do not ascribe to cultural standards of beauty is increasingly being interrogated in popular culture.

When fashion brand Diesel put out an open casting call for 'young culturally representative models', Jillian Mercado, a fashion blogger with disability, applied to the campaign. Her photograph features alongside 22 other 'unconventional' models in Diesel's 2014 Spring/Summer campaign. Mercado describes the campaign as 'so much bigger than an ad', commenting that 'anyone can wear Diesel – you don't have to be a supermodel, you don't have to be a millionaire, you can wear it no matter who you are and what you look like' (Mercado cited in White Sidell, 2014). Mercado's wheelchair holds a prominent position in several of the Diesel images.

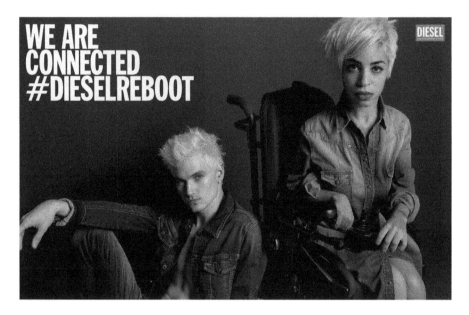

Figure 3.1   James Astronaut and Jillian Mercado in the Diesel 'We Are Connected' Campaign

Source: © Diesel. Photography by Inez and Vinoodh.

Mercado has received considerable media coverage since becoming a Diesel model. Most articles outline her 'surprise' at receiving a call back, given that she applied as a 'joke'. The language used to describe Mercado's – a long-time behind-the-scenes presence in fashion – arrival in front of the camera ranges from patronising, to celebratory, to 'fierce'. The discussion offers a snapshot into the plurality of fashion discourse and the way it constructs insiders and outsiders, as well as the different ways the beauty myth is invoked within this paradigm. Whereas Abercrombie and Fitch focus on the 'cool kids' and embrace the beauty myth, Diesel leverages the opposite ethos, those of the outsiders to attract customers. Diesel turns these outsiders into the 'cool kids'.

Laura Mulvey first coined the term 'to-be-looked-at-ness' in 1975 (see Mulvey, 1975). Mulvey argued that women were subject to a male gaze in Hollywood film. The camera becomes complicit in the domination of women by focusing on specific body parts, such as the breasts, face and legs, rather than the person as a whole. According to Mulvey, male characters drive the narratives and female characters are acted upon, they do not act. They are there simply to incite emotion and action from the male protagonist with whom the spectator identifies. As a result, spectators take on a male subjectivity regardless of their actual gender and sexuality. Like female characters, people with disability also connote 'to-be-looked-at-ness'; however, as Garland-Thomson (2001) explains, 'women are the proper object of the male gaze, while disabled people are the proper object of the stare'.

'Staring', Garland-Thomson explains, focuses on the disability and disregards the person as a whole, it 'registers the perception of difference and gives meaning to impairment by marking it as aberrant' (Garland-Thomson, 2002, p. 56). Garland-Thomson focuses her investigation of the stare on the way it is manipulated in popular photography. She argues that as previously acceptable spectacles of disability such as freak shows became unacceptable in the early twentieth century, photography 'enabled the social ritual of staring at disability to persist in an alternate form' (Garland-Thomson, 2002, p. 57). Photography began being used by a capitalist democracy to appropriate disability for specific purposes.

As the responsibility for people with disability shifted from the family and community towards science and medicine in the nineteenth century, people with disability began to be controlled by charity discourses. Snyder and Mitchell (2006) describe this shift as a process of 'cultural dislocation' and explain the way it subjugates people with disability by positioning disability as an individual concern and the charity of non-disabled people as morally uplifting (p. 39).

British social modellist David Hevey brings these concepts together in his book *The Creatures Time Forgot* to identify a medical, charity and impairment fixation with disability through an exposé of disability charity imagery. He argues that charity advertising constructs people with disability as tragic but brave 'creatures', objects of the camera's gaze. His is a political project designed to espouse a visual equivalent of 'rights not charity'. Garland-Thomson and Hevey note the significance of charity in shaping the public's perception of disability, particularly through the photographic gaze.

Staring at people with disability has been encouraged in popular culture from the earliest legends to freak shows to popular photography. While Garland-Thomson (2002) argues that wondrous, sentimental, exotic and realistic images of disability are all equally constructed to 'appropriate the disabled body for the purposes of constructing, instructing, or assuring some aspect of a putatively non-disabled viewer' (p. 59), people with disability and their allies are creating new insights and merging traditional and progressive media frames to offer different images, witness events and debate the potential for social change.

Elizabeth Wilson (2003) describes 'fashion' as essential to modernity and ironically positions it as a way to retain individualism in the face of the 'mass man' (p. 34). Fashion imagery and the cultural dislocation of charity discourses being applied to people with disability intersect when disability exotically appears within fashion imagery. The use of models with disability in fashion may 'mak[e] consumers feel good about buying from a company that is charitable toward the supposedly disadvantaged' (Garland-Thomson, 2002, p. 66). However, in general, fashion has focused on physical perfection in its definition of beauty.

This chapter draws upon memoir and media interviews to addresses the intersection between disability and the beauty myth from two different but related angles. My first aim is to consider the creation of a normative body through the beauty myth as a way to understand disability as socially and culturally situated. The second is to interrogate the way disability has been excluded from discourses of beauty. When considered in relation to the rigid parameters of beauty, ableism takes its place alongside other forms of social discrimination to reveal 'the cultural context surrounding and defining our bodies, not our bodies themselves, creates problems for us – and that this context rather than our bodies requires alteration' (Garland-Thomson, 1995, p. 4).

I begin the chapter by outlining Naomi Wolf's theory of the beauty myth to introduce social pressure to look and behave in certain ways experienced by women and people with disabilities. As Wolf (1993) argues, the beauty myth 'is always prescribing behaviour and not appearance' (p. 10). For women with disabilities, the pressure can be particularly intense because it is so much harder for these women to achieve the culturally prescribed notions of femininity However, as mentioned above, the notion that people with disability do not ascribe to cultural standards of beauty is increasingly being interrogated in popular culture. The next section of the chapter introduces John Clogston's media frames of disability to consider the differing approaches taken to the intersections between disability and the beauty myth and the ways the media continues to adopt an overly sympathetic tone despite opportunities for transgression. The chapter draws on case studies from fashion, reality television, pornography, the mainstream media and the blogosphere.

The Beauty Myth

While a number of feminists exposed beauty as a tool of the patriarchy during the 1970s, Naomi Wolf popularised the idea in *The Beauty Myth*. In her book, Wolf seeks to expose the way 'trivial concerns' related to body image and physical appearances were being used against women. She discerns a strong relationship between female liberation and female beauty, noting that where empowered women were breaking through the 'feminine mystique of domesticity', they were becoming re-enslaved to the beauty myth (Wolf, 2002, pp. 10–11). Wolf argues that unobtainable and rigid standards of beauty are being used to undo the gains of feminism. For Wolf, the beauty myth is not about beauty at all, it is about power and control. As she suggests, the 'gaunt yet full breasted Caucasian' (p. 2) who embodies the ideal in the mass media is rarely found in nature while all sorts of other bodies are.

The beauty myth creates a normative individual. 'Disabled' indeed describes many bodies that do not ascribe to cultural definitions of beauty through impairment, illness, injury, weight, age, deformity, scars or other features that do not pass as 'normal'. Further, according to Wolf (1993), the beauty myth proscribes female's primary social value as being 'the attainment of virtuous beauty' (p. 18). This social value is reinforced through the conflation of the ideal body with the normal body in the media and popular culture.

Nevertheless, recent theorisation in disability has begun focusing on the importance of discourses of beauty and the inclusion of disability within them. As Niall Richardson (2010) argues, disability studies must start to address the 'cult of contemporary beauty-ism' despite being attractive being lower on the list of needs than other disabling social issues (p. 172). Like Wolf, Richardson notes the ways beauty is positioned as trivial. However, as we shall see throughout this chapter, beauty is not a trivial issue, it is a heavily constructed agent of control and has real consequences for the lived experience of people with disability (see Shakespeare, 2000). Corporeal standards of normality are shifting such that 'our unmodified bodies are presented as unnatural and abnormal, whereas the surgically altered bodies are portrayed as normal and natural' (Garland-Thomson, 2011, p. 24). A clear example of this dissonance is the 'total body confidence' themed issue of *Self* magazine which featured Kelly Clarkson on the cover in 2009. The singer, who is known for her curvaceous body, was digitally slimmed down in her *Self* photos. The editors of *Self* justified their airbrushing of Clarkson claiming it was their job to 'inspire women to want to be their best' rather than present 'reality' (Danziger, 2009). Ironically, Clarkson is quoted on the cover of the magazine as saying 'stay true to you and everyone else will love you too'.

This example shows that the 'ideal' is increasingly being conflated with the norm in modern mass media, and that people are increasingly made to feel as though they have inadequate bodies. The tyranny of the beauty myth is that it affects different people in different ways, thus providing an opportunity to consider the cultural construction of disability. Normalcy and beauty are twin ideologies that render female and disabled bodies subject to infinite shaping to appeal to a socially constructed standard:

> The beautiful woman of the twenty-first century is sculpted surgically from
> top to bottom, generically neutral, all irregularities regularized, all particularities

expunged. She is thus nondisabled, deracialized and de-ethnicized. (Garland-Thomson, 2011, p. 24)

For Garland-Thomson, the image of impairment, such as nude photos of breast cancer survivors, can disrupt conventional understandings of beauty and integrate disability into feminist examinations of power relations. The images of Mercado in Diesel's *We are Connected* campaign also disrupt conventional understandings of beauty, particularly as they feature her wheelchair. The campaign follows the aesthetic introduced in Diesel's earlier Fall 2013 campaign which featured 'modern-day rebels, heroes and just cool people' found on social media such as Tumblr. Artistic director Nicola Formichetti describes his motivations for including models with disability, tattoos and facial hair:

I was looking for a rebellious attitude, which is so closely tied to denim ... The second campaign was much more about the group, the gang, the tribe, the community. The people got to us in different ways but they're connected visually, physically, mentally and denim is the thing that unites all of them. And that's the theme and the tag line – we are connected. (Formichetti cited in Karr, 2014)

Of Mercado he explains:

It's never easy for her to move from point A to point B, but she's totally fearless and has really been an inspiration to me ... You don't have to be a conventional model type to represent a brand. (Formichetti cited in White Sidell, 2014)

A number of articles about Mercado's participation in the Diesel campaign follow this inspirational theme and adopt the 'supercrip' media frame identified by John Clogston (1994) and discussed later in the chapter. Clogston differentiated media coverage of disability into progressive and traditional frames, finding that sometimes articles moved between both contexts. For example, Riam Dean was often described as a student or a sales assistant in news coverage. She was a multifaceted person with legitimate political grievances (progressive). Yet unnecessary medical details were introduced and she was often constructed within the supercrip discourse (traditional) (see Pidd, 2009). Similarly, although the *Daily Mail* outlines Jillian Mercado's college-level education and difficulties with New York's public transport system, stereotypes of disability are invoked when Mercado is strangely described as 'more cheerful' than her fellow students (White Sidell, 2014).

Disabling the Beauty Myth

In the 2002 republication of *The Beauty Myth*, Wolf recalls the feedback she received from numerous beautiful women 'who looked like fashion models' who believed they did not meet the ideal. These women 'admitted to knowing, from the time they could consciously think, that the ideal was someone tall, thin, white, and blond. A face without pores, asymmetry, or flaws, someone wholly "perfect", and someone who they felt, in one way or another, they were not' (Wolf, 2002, p. 1). Angela Rockwood, star and producer of the reality television series *Push Girls* articulates this disconnect in her comparison of her approach to body image pre- and post-paralysis:

> I was that gym rat that was in the gym three hours every single day. I had almost the perfect 10 body, and I still struggled to make sure I was perfect. And then all of a sudden I get into a car accident, and here I am, my body's atrophied, I have very thin arms, I've got my little "quad" belly, and my legs ... I lost all my muscle tone. But the funny thing is, I look at my body now, and I love who I am! I embrace my body now. I'm so comfortable in my skin. When I was walking and had a great body, I wasn't comfortable in my skin. (Rockwood cited in Kuster, 2012)

Rockwood, who was a model prior to becoming quadriplegic and is shown attempting to re-enter the industry throughout *Push Girls,* thus positions her disability as an opportunity to opt out of the beauty myth to a certain degree (Carlson, 2013). However, notions of beauty and glamour continue to pervade this show, a characteristic that has been both criticised and celebrated.

Indeed, scenes within *Push Girls* illustrate the continuing relevance of beauty, fashion and sexuality to women with disability. For example, in episode 3, Tiphany and Auti – who are between 10 and 20 years post-disablement – take newly disabled Chelsie shopping for high heels. Tiphany explains that wearing heels 'makes you feel like a woman again'. Auti positions the shoes as an important step in Chelsie's recovery and her moves towards independence. Auti will 'bless' her the shoes but Chelsie must figure out a way to get them on her feet herself. Chelsie explains that the experience has taught her that 'you can be beautiful and in a wheelchair'. This scene has been heavily criticised for perpetuating the beauty myth and suggesting people with disability embrace 'form over function'. As Lisa Holms argues:

> What turns me off most is their obsession with appearances – form over function. Not wearing leg straps so your foot ends up scraping on the pavement under you? Wearing HIGH HEELS? (Lisa Holm comment on THR Staff, 2012)

The topic has been previously covered within disability-specific publications such as the *New Mobility* magazine which considered the importance of discourses of beauty – specifically shoes – to women who have acquired a disability sense of self. The insights of a number of women with a variety of impairments reveal the operation of the beauty myth and its presence in adjusting to life and identity with disability. Some describe liberation in casting off the confines of uncomfortable shoes while others reject the notion of giving up on fashion despite the added pain of heels etc. The idea of transitional shoes associated with illness and rehabilitation also emerges as a particularly harrowing experience:

> Then came a spinal cord injury, hospital-issue Stryker boots and sparkling white oversized hightops for rehab. Looking back at the few photos I have of myself from that time – with my custom-cut halo vest T-shirts, baggy sweats and blinding white shoes – I think it's no surprise that my self image was shot. This was not a good look. Certainly not self-assured, certainly not sexy. With a Foley, a Theravac and a package of powdered gloves, I looked ready to wheel into the gimp sunset with only my white shoes to light my way. (McGowen, 2011)

BBC blogger Disability Bitch brings the beauty myth and concepts of female disablement together when she quips:

> I've always been a supporter of high heels. Think about it. As types of footwear go, they at least put disabled and non-disabled women on a level, as they render even the most Amazonian and able female slightly mobility impaired. (Disability Bitch, 2008)

Pam Matteson is similarly quoted in the *New Mobility* article:

> My shoe choices over the years have been based on fashion fads, not on ignoring or disliking my feet. My feet are probably the most aesthetically pleasing and intact part of my gimped-out body, so why not glorify them? They are not atrophied like my legs, pouchy like my belly, or bony like my butt, but perfectly smooth and better looking than any AB's [sic]. I do think that what you wear on your feet is a reflection of your self-esteem. Shoes are just part of the whole "put together" image I am out to convey. I don't see any reason I have to wear dumpy grandma shoes. I am a vibrant, self-assured woman who uses a wheelchair – not a wheelchair that has a woman in it. The woman comes first. (Matteson cited in McGowen, 2011)

While Disability Bitch's article highlights the way women are disabled by fashion and the ways women with disability are frequently excluded from participation in this arena, Matteson's insight reveals the continuing importance of fashion and beauty to some women with disability (although it is interesting to note that others cited within the article disagree). Even as the older women in *Push Girls* instruct Chelsie that heels will help her regain her sense of self as feminine, the irony of the claim is highlighted in practical terms because the scene immediately follows Tiphany's admission that she does not always use foot straps and has injured her feet as a result.

Whereas Wolf's feminist critique sought to reveal the way women are entrapped and oppressed through the beauty myth, Michelle Fine and Adrienne Asch observe that, 'women with disability have not been "trapped" by many of the social expectations that feminists have challenged' (1988 cited in Schriempf, 2001, p. 54). Ellen Stohl, the first woman with disability to pose for *Playboy*, actively sought out the beauty myth as part of a wider project on reclaiming her feminine identity following paralysis. Stohl explains her reason for seeking out the soft core pornographic magazine, 'they focus on the ideal image of a woman. If I can achieve that, I can be anything in between' (Stohl cited in Smith, 1988).

Ellen Stohl Poses for Playboy: Applauded and Condemned

In 1985, two years after sustaining a spinal cord injury, aspiring model and college student Ellen Stohl wrote to Hugh Hefner of *Playboy* suggesting the magazine feature a model with disability in recognition that people with disability are sexual:

> sexuality is the hardest thing for disabled persons to hold onto. Not to say that they are not capable, but rather that society's emphasis on perfection puts this definitive damper on self-esteem. Well, I believe it is time to show society the real story. Anyone can be sexy. (Stohl cited in Cooper, 1995)

While Hefner situates *Playboy*'s decision to feature Stohl as part of a broader project of reversing the view that human sexuality is dirty (see Cooper, 1995), as Quinlan and Bates (2008) caution, 'sexualized images may create a new beauty myth to which individuals with disability must aspire' (p. 75). They note that those who can pass as able-bodied, or most closely resemble it, are considered the most attractive.

Stohl received extensive media coverage and was described in the *New York Times* as meeting the 'bosomy, cellulite-free [standard of] attractiveness' required of *Playboy* models (Cummings, 1987). In keeping with the playmates' 'themes', Stohl was represented in *Playboy* as a student in a student's apartment rather than as a person with disability. While there were photographs of her in her wheelchair wearing clothes, the sexualised imagery does not suggest any physical impairment. Stohl is quoted in an article published in the *LA Times* as preferring the sexualised imagery because 'her body seems to be nearly perfect' (Smith, 1988).

In a series of media interviews and within the *Playboy* article itself, Stohl describes experiencing a loss of sexuality when she became disabled. She explains that people began viewing her as an asexual child, rather than a woman. The issues Stohl raises in and through *Playboy* reveal the ways women with disability must first establish the existence of sexuality before they can assert a feminist project of control over it:

> Especially since my accident, I've felt that sexuality is the very essence of who we are … and if somebody or something takes away your sexuality, you don't know who you are or where you fit in … [After the crash] I was a child again, and people treated me as such, not as a woman … I was really lucky in that two orderlies in the hospital harassed me relentlessly – tried to pull my sheets off and stuff. They treated me like a woman. . . . It's funny – if I sit in my wheelchair, a lot of guys don't want to approach me, because they don't know how. But if I'm on a barstool, I'll be ripped off and asked to dance. And I'm not doing anything different; I'm just sitting in a different chair. . . . I suppose there'll be those women's libbers who say, "I don't want to be seen as just a sex object". No, of course you don't want to be seen as just that. But would you want that taken away from you? (Stohl 1987 cited in Schriempf, 2001, p. 56)

Stohl's interview simultaneously reveals a problematic sexist attitude and a problem in the way women with disability are viewed. While feminist discourse asserts a woman's right to make their own decisions about their own sexuality, disabled women are frequently believed to have no sexuality at all.

In a 1988 keynote address to the Southern Connecticut State University Women's Studies Conference entitled 'Fulfilling Possibilities: Women and Girls with Disabilities', Nadina LaSpina postulates that the negative impacts of this loss of sexuality include a lack of access to sex education and health care. She recalls her own reaction to Stohl's appearance in *Playboy*, 'disabled women have been fighting for the right to be attractive and sexual, at times acting in ways that would make our feminist sisters frown. I remember that as a feminist I was appalled when Ellen Stohl (a gorgeous quadriplegic woman) posed for Playboy. But as a Disabled woman, I understood and fully identified with her need to flaunt her sexiness' (LaSpina, 1988). Stohl herself similarly argued:

> I wasn't taking off my clothes for men. I didn't pose for *Playboy* to please men. I posed for *Playboy* to discover my own sexuality, to celebrate that part of me that was stripped away by a disability because our society doesn't put sexuality and disability together. (Stohl cited in Cooper, 1995)

Stohl explains her approach to *Playboy* was motivated by a need to 'regain my identity as a woman' (Stohl cited in Harris, 2002). While *Playboy* editors were concerned they would be accused of exploiting the disabled to get attention and sell more copies of the magazine, *Playboy* associate editor Kate Nolan explains that the feature on Stohl 'probably didn't sell one extra magazine' (Nolan cited in Smith, 1988). The issue featured an eight-page photo layout and an accompanying article which outlined the debate among *Playboy* staff about whether to feature a model with disability. Associate editor Barbara Nellis outlines the types of concerns highlighted by *Playboy* staff as the issue went to print:

> This is precisely the kind of attention that Playboy doesn't need. The only thing that people are going to say is, "Have you seen what Playboy is doing? Girls in wheelchairs." The argument in favor of running the pictorial is that the editorial copy that runs with the photographs is sensitively written. But be serious. There is not a horribly big leap between this and real scuzz exploitation. If Playboy wanted to seriously discuss the issue of sexuality and the disabled, we could have run a portrait of the woman's face and an essay. This is very difficult to explain and defend. The average person will see it and say, "Boy, Playboy must be in some kind of terrible trouble." (Barbara Nellis cited in Greene, 1987)

Other staff members expressed concern that *Playboy* would be considered 'bad taste' for 'fetishizing' a 'cripple' (see Greene, 1987). Editorial director Arthur Kretchmer explains his reasons for deciding to run the images, despite concerns about how the public would react:

> We all so easily dehumanize people ... We categorize people because it's easy. We categorize people in wheelchairs as "cripples," and we all get on with our lives and forget about them ... I may be naive, but I don't see [the images of Stohl] as exploitation. The word "exploitation" comes up in other contexts when people criticize Playboy, but in this case I think we're on the side of the angels ... I think we are honoring Ellen Stohl's faith in us. We are allowing her to be whole – to be sexual – and I think it is a wonderful tribute to Playboy that we are the magazine to which she wrote. (Arthur Kretchmer cited in Greene, 1987)

The eight-page *Playboy* spread similarly generated significant discussion among disability activists, particularly around the erasure of Stohl's disability within the sexualised images. Stohl's urging that *Playboy* consider her a 'sexual object' rather than an 'asexual object' (Stohl cited in Willig Levy, 1998) was discussed extensively in the disability community. For example, the disability advocacy magazine *The Disability Rag* debated the issue across three consecutive issues. Indeed the debate went beyond Stohl herself to consider the broader context of disability and sexuality.

Disability advocate Chava Willig Levy lists the 'controversy' as a significant moment in the history of the Independent Living Movement. She labels the connection between *Playboy* and liberation as 'considered dubious by feminists, controversial by most others' and outlines the ways both disability-specific publications such as the *Disability Rag* and mainstream media highlighted the ironies of the pictorial which seemed to separate disability and sexuality in the actual nude photographs of Stohl (Willig Levy, 1998).

Michael Stein connects Stohl's purported reclamation of sexuality with other examples in popular culture such as sexual tropes in film (e.g. *Coming Home, Born on the Fourth of July* and *The Waterdance*), Ray Charles's assertion that he may be blind but he is not dead and therefore still knows beautiful women (specifically his backup singers the 'beautiful Rayettes') and a John Callahan cartoon of a man in a wheelchair being escorted to a hospital exit by four heavily pregnant nurses captioned 'Handicapped People Don't Have Sex' (Stein, 1994). Stohl, Willig Levy and Stein therefore argue that the *Playboy* issue represented a significant moment in potentially shifting social views of people with disability as asexual and unattractive.

However, critiques remained that the pictures of Stohl in *Playboy* did not advance the disability rights agenda. Kate Nolan is on record as agreeing with a number of these critiques. She questioned what *Playboy* was trying to achieve by photographing Stohl as though she was 'just like everybody else' (Cummings, 1987), that is without her wheelchair. The images thus suggest a separation of Stohl's sexuality and her disability. Her disability is visible in the images of her day to day life, socialising at a fraternity and participating in a martial arts class. It is, however, erased in the soft core porn. Nolan argued that *Playboy* was making an empty statement; '[we wouldn't] run pictures of someone who was really, seriously deformed' (Nolan cited in Greene, 1987). Arthur Kretchmer conceded some agreement here:

> I agree with Kate Nolan that this would all be different if Ellen Stohl was terribly disfigured. In that case, we would be putting on what would be called a freak show. We're not doing that. (Arthur Kretchmer cited in Greene, 1987)

Kretchner's assertion suggests that, despite featuring Stohl, the magazine still continued to disassociate disability and sexuality, reinforcing the alternative beauty myth that Quinlan and Bates (2008) caution against. Irving Zola, who was editor of the journal *Disability Studies Quarterly* at the time of Stohl's *Playboy* issue, argued that the photographs 'reinforced precisely what Stohl has complained about: "society's emphasis on perfection." They've satisfied their own demand that Stohl look like everyone else by creating the illusion that she does'. He suggested instead they photograph Stohl naked in her wheelchair (Zola cited in Smith, 1988).

Hugh Hefner explains why they elected not to include her wheelchair:

> The decision was consistent with not associating her disability. It is down that road that takes you into a exploitative kinky type of thing. In other words, a part of what this is all about is her disability and the chair began to define who she was, and that she was not perceived as a human sexual being. (Hefner cited in Cooper, 1995)

Nevertheless Levy saw potential in the issue. She concludes her discussion of the ironic alliance by 'looking on the bright side':

> … one could conclude that Ms. Stohl's feature shattered the myth that disability and deformity must go hand-in-hand. The next step, which hopefully will occur in life rather than Playboy, is to demonstrate that deformity, like disability, has no devaluing effect on sexual appeal. (Willig Levy, 1998)

The debate that raged among the *Playboy* staff and within the disability community in the lead up to and aftermath of Stohl's *Playboy* pictorial reveal that people did not know how to represent disability in the context of this particular paradigm of sexuality in 1987. Although two further disabled models, both amputees (Jennifer Krum in 2005 and Debbie Van der Putten in 2008) have posed for *Playboy*, arguably, we still don't. While the Stohl images may be considered dubious (see Garland-Thomson, 2011 for a good discussion), the dialogue it elicited reveal the ways people use popular culture to make meaning in their own lives and the significance of popular culture in eliciting discussion about disability inclusion.

The June 1987 issue of *Playboy* represents a significant moment in disability popular culture. The images of Stohl continue to be discussed within critical disability studies and Stohl herself continues to receive mainstream media attention. The ongoing coverage of Ellen Stohl also reveals the way many find it difficult to accept the socially constructed aspects of disability and instead adopt an 'overly sympathetic' response (see Garland-Thomson, 1995, p. 302). While Stohl claims to have selected *Playboy* because 'any other magazine would have published a clichéd "triumph-over-tragedy" story' (Smith, 1988), continuing media coverage over an almost 30-year period has embraced an overly sympathetic media framework at times invoking a disability as inspirational paradigm.

Twenty five years after posing for *Playboy*, Stohl continued to focus on the separation between her sexuality and wheelchair outlining her motivations for posing in *Playboy* as making the statement 'Look at me! I am a woman more than I am a wheelchair and you need to see that about me' (Stohl cited in Magers, 2011). She notes the continuing significance of her *Playboy* photos, framing changing embodiment as something we will all surely deal with, if we become old enough: 'disability is not going away ... and if we can't deal with the changes in our bodies and the changes in our physique, whether it's from aging or catastrophic injury, we limit what we can do' (Stohl cited in Magers, 2011). However, contrary to Stohl's initial intention, the article in which these quotes appear frame Stohl as an inspiration, albeit a sexy inspiration.

Media Frames

In 1990 John S. Clogston examined the language used, issues covered and overall portrayal of disability in 363 newspaper articles about physical disability. He also interviewed reporters about their attitudes. He found two models through which newspapers covered disability – traditional and progressive. Traditional approaches focused on disability as an individual's problem and society's role as only to 'cure or maintain', and could be further delineated into three frames:

> The Medical Model: Emphasis is on the individual's physical disability as an illness. The individual is portrayed as dependent on health professionals for cures or maintenance. Also included in this model are stories that focus primarily on the physical aspects of an individual's disability
> Supercrip Model: As in the medical model, individuals are focused on because of the physical characteristics of their disability. Individuals are portrayed either as "superhuman" because of physical feats (e.g. rock climbing paraplegics) or "amazing" because they function "normally, in spite of their disabilities"
> Social Pathology or Economic Model: Individuals with disabilities are portrayed as disadvantaged clients who look to the state or society for economic support, which is considered a gift, not a right. The individuals are portrayed as passive recipients of government or private economic support. (Clogston, 1994, p. 47)

By comparison, progressive approaches locate the problem of disability within inaccessible environments (physical, social and occupational) and people's prejudicial attitudes. Clogston notes the progressive model adopts two frames:

> Minority/Civil Rights: the person with disability is shown as member of a minority group dealing with legitimate political grievances, usually involved in disability rights political activities, actively demanding political change

Cultural Pluralism: The person with disability is considered a multifaceted individual whose disability is just one aspect of many. No undue attention is paid to the disability. The individual is portrayed as are others without disabilities. (Clogston, 1994, p. 47)

Traditional approaches focused on the individual's differences, whereas progressive stories focused on society's inability to deal with difference. Clogston also noted that sometimes articles would move between traditional and progressive approaches. Clogston concluded that newspaper coverage of disability was neither wholly traditional, nor wholly progressive, and that there was still much work to do to improve coverage and 'move toward full participation in society' (p. 51).

While Clogston's frames are still an important part of disability theorisation and others, most notably Beth Haller, have built on them in the intervening years, the internet and World Wide Web has created a new form of democratic publication that also provides insight into the cultural construction of disability. While I will discuss this so-called 'new media' in greater depth in Chapter 8, for now I point to the opportunity for people with and without disability to publish articles on blogs and correct already published materials through comments functions on blogs and forums.

Bruns and Jacobs (2006) describe ordinary people's participation on blogs, online journals and de facto news sites as a shift from production to produsage. Produsage is the interchangeable consumptive and productive mode of participant engagement with interactive environments. Media frames continue to be seen even in produsage; however, the opportunity for a merging of traditional and progressive approaches is encouraged as people with more and less experience with disability come together in online spaces to discuss its cultural construction.

The Veneer of Perfection

As part of International Day of Persons with Disabilities celebrations, Pro Infirmis, an organisation for the disabled, created and then displayed disabled mannequins on Zurich's Bahnhofstrasse. Mannequins with scoliosis, brittle bone disease, shortened limbs and malformed spines were positioned between 'perfect mannequins', all modelling the latest fashions.

A four minute video entitled *Because Who is Perfect?* captures the process of producing these mannequins and was released online. The video begins with close up shots of 'perfect' mannequin body parts – a flat stomach, lean legs and a muscular torso. Then, people with visible disabilities begin arriving at an artist's studio where their bodies are measured and an artist/photographer explains they will use these measurements to create mannequins whose bodies are 'different'. A number of craftspeople then begin altering shop mannequins so that they more closely resemble these disabled bodies. One of the participants in the video comments that she thinks it will 'be really difficult to make a copy of this', highlighting the idea that, unlike shop mannequins, people are all different and can not be cut from a mould. The video then goes on to illustrate the painstaking process these craftspeople take to modify the mannequins.

The disabled body takes on a vastly different meaning within the montage of measuring, cutting and rebuilding within *Because Who Is Perfect*. The disabled people come to look like works of art rather than less than perfect bodies. As the mannequins are revealed to the disabled models they express pride in their bodies – the woman who questioned whether the disabled mannequins could really be created commented that 'it is special to see yourself like this when you usually can't look at yourself in the mirror'. The mannequins are then displayed wearing the latest fashions in shop windows and passer-bys with and without disability look at the mannequins with curiosity. The video ends with the words 'Because Who is Perfect? Get Closer'.

Following the YouTube posting of the video, a number of posters comment on the emotive nature of the video and actively discuss the effects, both positive and negative, of merging discourses of fashion, beauty and disability in an attempt to normalise disability. This post by DreamBelief, who identifies as a person with disability, captures both the emotion provoked by the video and the ensuing discussion, and explains the importance of including disability within beauty:

> As someone with disabilities, and with family and friends with disabilities as well, this video makes me very happy. I do not like when people suggest that just because there is something wrong with us physically then we are not beautiful and that we have to see our physical disability in a negative way. I, and many I know, prefer to see our physical imperfections in a positive light and show people that it's not something to be scared of, just something a bit different to them. (DreamBelief comment on Pro Infirmus, 2013)

In addition to the YouTube discussion, both the video and the mannequins themselves have been covered by a number of media outlets. While a significant proportion of journalists and online commenters or forum participants recognise the event as a 'publicity stunt' designed to feel good about the disabled on one special day each year, producerly concepts of beauty are identified, as this comment on Gawker Media website Jezebel demonstrates:

> While this still feels like a publicity stunt, I seriously don't care. I don't think most people realize how important it is to actually see different body types. When all you see around you are photo-shopped models and impossibly thin mannequins,

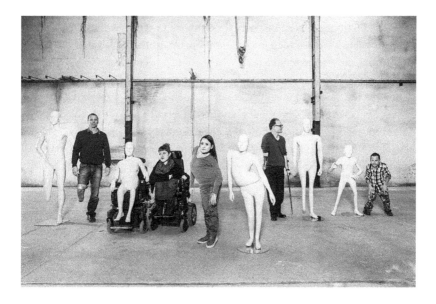

Figure 3.2 Because Who Is Perfect?

Source: Pro Infirmis 2013 Campaign. © www.proinfirmis.ch.

you start to internalize that concept as "normal". The structure of the human body is incredibly complex, with an infinite number of configurations, all of which can be seen as beautiful when viewed through a compassionate lens. And I feel that familiarity breeds compassion. It is hard to "other" the familiar. I wish these mannequins were in every store across the freaking planet, with one caveat: not all of them need to be white. Seriously. People of color exist, fashion industry. I love what you are doing here, but you need to take it a step farther. (beevomlt comment on Stewart, 2013)

Although the majority of discussion has been overwhelmingly positive, an article published on *The Sociological Cinema* raises several negative points for discussion:

These new mannequins of unfamiliar proportions stop passersby in their tracks and encourage them to reconsider the types of bodies that belong in storefronts, but while the video captures a useful disruption in the usual discourse on bodies, in my view it fails to truly provoke onlookers to reassess their casual assumptions about bodies as either working or broken, and as either worthy or unworthy of representation. No, the video leaves this binary cultural logic unscathed. For instance, one finds in the video that "able-bodied" mannequins are the clean slate from which "disabled" mannequins are born. There is a manufacturing

51

montage that puts to rest any radical doubts as to whether these two species of mannequin have anything in common. Finally, when displayed in the Zurich storefronts, the altered mannequins remain almost hermetically sealed from the original mannequins, which have been scuttled away for the event. To truly "get closer," as the video commands us to do, I think it is important to collapse this casual, Manichean distinction between the able-bodied and the disabled. A truly radical video might instead show the old mannequins displayed alongside the new ones, and the displays would be left in place long after the International Day of Persons with Disabilities was over. (*The Sociological Cinema*, 2014)

The Sociological Cinema therefore encourages viewers to really 'get closer' by questioning the binary logic of disabled versus not. Binary oppositions attempt to create an either/or environment that demarcates people into particular categories. The video presents a continuum of beauty and encourages viewers to question what perfection is. Just as people with disability do not fit into cultural standards of perfection, the majority of viewers would not look like a shop front mannequin either, if that is indeed the definition of perfection in any case. The video presents an in-between space of perfect v not perfect.

Breast cancer survivors have also utilised the photographic medium to disrupt conventional images of beauty. During the 1980s an anti-breast cancer campaign featured a shoot of women who had undergone mastectomies. The images intertextually referenced Victoria Secret catalogues and Calvin Klein advertisements. Rosemarie Garland-Thomson has covered these images extensively in her work on staring to argue that they challenge the, 'representational practices that make everyday erotic spectacles of women's breasts while erasing the fact of the amputated breast' (Garland-Thomson, 2011, p. 26).

More recently, the photographic exhibition and website *Under the Red Dress* seeks to go beneath the veneer of perfection, to force contemporary Australia to literally and figuratively look at breast cancer. The first image is of a conventionally attractive blonde wearing a vibrant red dress. Following the conventions of fashion imagery, she embodies a familiar 'to-be-looked-at-ness' and, as we are invited to look beneath the red dress, the visual conventions of beauty are ruptured as her body reveals a double mastectomy and a number of scars. The project's description touches on many of the issues discussed throughout this chapter:

The version of ourselves that we unwittingly portray to the world. It's desirable, strong, beautiful and everybody admires it. This veneer has been constructed by the very fabric of the societies in which we live. The ideologies we grow up with, what's acceptable, what's not. We all want to belong, to be accepted and so we feel we must be a certain way, and we fit in because it's easier. And at first it might feel like it really is. So we cling to this veneer as if life depends upon it, and in so doing may feel the need to hide what's going on underneath.

Photographer Nadia Mascot and model Beth Whaanga sought to expose the impacts these performative aspects of humanness and femininity have on people who don't fit the 'norm'. They go on to highlight the temporariness of a desirable, strong and beautiful body with the assertion that life is unpredictable and we could all, at any moment be affected by illness, injury or another body-altering event that could make us look and feel different. Within its wider project of encouraging breast self-examination, *Under the Red Dress* urges people to reconsider what beauty is and who possesses it:

> But what if life deals us an unexpected blow? Sickness. Accident. Abuse. War. Birth defects. We then bare the body-altering scars that not only make us look different, but perhaps make us see ourselves differently too. For those of us who find ourselves physically scarred by life's events, we can easily slip into this idea that we are not beautiful at all. What is beauty anyway? Let's redefine.

Through an interrogation of humanness, survival and beauty, the pictures critique a culture of passing, of pretending these things do not happen.

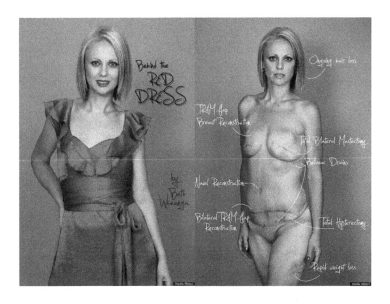

Figure 3.3   Beth Whaanga poses for 'Under the Red Dress'
Source: © Nadia Mascot.

However, when Whaanga posted the images on her Facebook wall with the below warning, over 100 people unfriended her.

> These images are confronting and contain topless material. They are not in anyway meant to be sexual. The aim of this project is to raise awareness for breast cancer. If you find these images offensive please hide them from your feed.
>
> Each day we walk past people. These individuals appear normal but under their clothing sometimes their bodies tell a different story. Nadia Mascot and I aim to find others who are willing to participate in our project so that we might show others that cancer effects everyone. The old and the young, age does not matter, self-examination is vital. It can happen to you. (Whaanga cited in Sparrow, 2014)

The negative reaction to these images reveals that perhaps people feel more comfortable in their ignorance, that they would prefer to walk past the people who appear normal (maybe even beautiful) and not be disrupted by the presence of difference. They do not want to know it 'can happen to them'. The photos have since been blocked under Facebook's 'pornographic' rules. Simi Linton (1998) describes this as passing and suggests it is both an act of cultural survival and an exhausting cultural expectation to live up to. Seen in the context of Linton's observations, this mass unfriending reveals the ways our culture 'insists upon, reinforces, or otherwise shames the individual into [passing]' (Linton, 1998, p. 20).

The unfriending, however, was countered by an overly sympathetic media response which invoked the features of Clogston's supercrip media frame. For example, Whaanga was headlined as 'more than brave' on popular culture site MamaMia and discussed on Twitter as inspirational, a battler, brave and heartfelt. Whaanga herself spoke back using Facebook and described herself as a 'breast cancer presenter' ("Was this woman's heartfelt facebook post really offensive?", 2014). While the people who unfriended her were heavily criticised, the majority of the news sites did not feature the nude *Under the Red Dress* images and instead cropped the photos to show only Whaanga's face.

Conclusion

Increasingly narrow parameters of beauty and normality offer an opportunity for all people, regardless of whether they have a disability or impairment, to reflect on the ways bodies are marginalised according to seemingly arbitrary cultural values. Naomi Wolf called this the beauty myth and outlined the way it demanded certain behaviour and bodily intervention to re-enslave women who had become liberated through feminism. Since the first print of Wolf's book, the beauty myth has intensified and the ideal is becoming increasingly conflated with the norm. We have seen how critical disability theorists such as Susan Wendell and Rosemarie Garland-Thomson have continued the debate, revealing the way this further impacts people with disability.

The disabled body is rejected and feared and subject to medical and welfare constructions. Media framing has been complicit in constructing disabled bodies as being unable to work and in need of medical intervention. However, as the exposés of Dean's firing, Clarkson's air brushing, and the unfriending of Whaanga reveal, the media is also a powerful agent of change.

The other side to this story is that people with disability are considered outside discourses of beauty and sexuality. As Fine and Asch argue, women with disability in particular are not subject to the same social expectations that have disempowered women in general. Yet the insights of Disability Bitch, the *Push Girls*, the women with disability interviewed in *New Mobility*, and Ellen Stohl reveal that this exclusion may serve as another site of cultural disablement.

For example, this chapter discussed Ellen Stohl posing in *Playboy* as a key moment in disability popular culture. While the images are largely considered problematic – and I concede here are not enough in and of themselves to change the view that people with disability are unattractive and asexual – they served as an opportunity for discussion in both disability-specific publications and within the mainstream media.

While Stohl's images are largely criticised for reinforcing the beauty myth and positioning Stohl as indistinguishable from a non-disabled centrefold, the discussion continues as images and videos of clearly disabled, injured and impaired bodies have been distributed online with a view to encourage viewers to reassess constructs of beauty. Where Diesel's *We are Connected* campaign featuring images of Mercado attempts to draw in those people positioned as 'outsiders' by the fashion industry, *Because Who is Perfect* encourages viewers to reassess their own view of people with disability, and *Under the Red Dress* both critiques a culture of passing and, perhaps unintentionally, reveals the way people cling to it.

Chapter 4
Spaces of Cultural Mediation: The Science Fiction Cinema of the Third Stage of Disability

In Andrew Nichol's *Gattaca* (1997) Vincent Freeman, a man with an undesirable genetic makeup, dreams of becoming an astronaut. In order to achieve his goal he must assume the identity of a person with superior genes, whose conception was genetically engineered. Jerome Morrow, a former athlete who became a paraplegic following a failed suicide attempt, sells Vincent his genetic profile, blood and DNA to use in the numerous genetic tests required to succeed in the workforce of this futuristic world. As Vincent takes on Jerome's identity, he is easily accepted into the Gattaca astronaut program but, when a mission director is murdered days before Vincent is due to fly to Saturn and his 'inferior' DNA is discovered at the scene, a heavy police presence jeopardises his future. Despite the investigation and several close calls, the film ends with Vincent flying into space and Jerome killing himself in an incinerator Vincent had used throughout the film to dispose of his 'invalid' DNA.

Joss Whedon's feature film *Serenity* (2005) is based on his short-lived television series *Firefly* (2002). Set 500 years in the future, both tell the story of the crew of Captain Mal Reynold's 'firefly-class' transport ship *Serenity* as they travel the outer galaxy doing both legal and illegal transport jobs. Teenager River Tam, who was smuggled onto the ship by her brother Dr Simon Tam, is a psychic child prodigy wanted by the government. Her behaviour, which has been likened to characteristics of autism (Bernardin, 2008), is a source of ire for some members of the crew who prefer to go about their business unnoticed. They begrudge Mal's insistence on protecting her. While at the conclusion of *Firefly* it is unclear what River's affliction actually is, throughout *Serenity* it becomes apparent that her brain was altered at the private school she attended, the Alliance Academy – a government experiment in creating the perfect assassin posing as a private school for talented youngsters. While there, River was subject to medical experimentation and brainwashing and, as a result, acquired telepathic powers but lost her ability to regulate her emotions. Throughout the television series and film, River is often considered a burden rather than asset by the other characters, yet she is extremely logical and is even able to anticipate attacks against the ship and crew. *Serenity* concludes with her serving as Mal's co-pilot.

Blade Runner also interrogates what happens when corporations attempt to manipulate human life for the purpose of colonisation and manual labour. Humanoids known as replicants are developed for slave labour. They are described as 'superior in strength and agility, and at least equal in intelligence, to the genetic engineers who created them' in the introductory titles to the film. Following a bloody mutiny, the replicants are declared illegal on earth and bounty hunters such as the character Deckard are engaged to track and 'retire' (kill) them. However, as he proceeds, the emotion which is said to differentiate humans from replicants becomes more difficult to decipher, and the viewer is ultimately left wondering whether Deckard himself is a replicant.

These examples could be expanded to include numerous films in which characters with disability feature in major and minor roles to offer a critique of the way the information age and technological progress may create disabling environments. These narratives are set in and beyond the third stage of disability as identified by Vic Finkelstein (1980), whereby people with disability are socially integrated as long as they are participating in the workforce. With these films also offering the opportunity to work in lucrative black markets, characters with disability are neither excluded from the workforce nor expected to make use of technologies that are not suitably adapted for their bodies.

Disability film criticism, which has historically focused on social-realist genres, has recently turned its attention towards science fiction cinema (Allan, 2013; Bérubé, 2005; Cheyne, 2009; Johnson, 2002; McReynolds, 2013), a genre which interrogates the 'issue of humanness' and associated themes of difference (Neale, 2000, p. 102). Significantly, science fiction takes up the concerns introduced in early disability criticism that sought to advance an understanding of disability as exclusion from the workforce (Finkelstein, 1981). In addition, we now exist in an era of medical and scientific research where typical science fiction narratives around medical enhancements of the human body and curing physical impairment could become a reality (see Naam, 2012).

This chapter critically examines the representation of disability in cinema to problematise the identification of ableist stereotypes. The chapter begins by outlining the trajectory of disability-film analysis as it moves through several stages – from social model stereotypes to a cultural analysis of the problem body – using the social-realist film *Million Dollar Baby*. The chapter then moves to introduce the importance of science fiction genres such as cyberpunk and post-cyberpunk as they advance core theories of the social model of disability. Both critical and optimistic disability readings of the films *Gattaca* and *Avatar* will be used to offer a producerly mode of disability film analysis that takes into account both social and cultural models of disability.

Disability Film Analysis: Narrative Codes

Cinematic codes assist in making stories easier to understand for audiences. They refer to everything that is seen and heard within a shot as well as camera angles and editing. In analysing these codes, it is important to pay attention to what is emphasised, omitted and valued. Disability is rarely valued – it is often omitted from leading roles and is emphasised for particular reasons, usually to elicit an emotional response. Clint Eastwood's 2004 film *Million Dollar Baby* about Maggie – a strong willed female boxer reaching the heights of her sport, succeeding in spite of gender prejudice only to experience massive personal tragedy in the form of disablement – garnered attention from both disability activists and academics when it was released. The film clearly demonstrates the way narratives codes work – disability is not valued, and is both omitted and emphasised for different reasons.

Despite refusing to accept socially imposed limitations regarding gender throughout the film, Maggie does not even seek out rehabilitation when she acquires disability. Her impairment is emphasised to communicate the shifting characterisation of her trainer Frankie from a hard, uncaring chauvinist to a loving father figure. Frankie's mercy killing of Maggie at the end of the film illustrates the ultimate omission of disability. As Davis explains in his critique of the film, *Million Dollar Baby* constructs disability as a personal tragedy rather than a political struggle:

> … the feisty girl who would stop at nothing to fight in the ring, who tells her greedy, hick family to bugger off, strangely changes character and becomes someone who gives up her ghost rather quickly – even refusing Frankie's offer of sending her to college (his one passing attempt to alleviate her despair). (Davis, 2005)

Davis locates the problematic representation of disability in *Million Dollar Baby* as a continuation of director Clint Eastwood's disability prejudice. In 1997 a wheelchair user filed an ADA complaint against Eastwood because the doors and restrooms in his hotel the Mission Ranch Inn were inaccessible. Eastwood later described the requirement to provide reasonable accommodations for disabled patrons to his hotel as 'a form of extortion' (Davis, 2005).

Stereotypes

Stereotypes offer a grossly simplified version of life. This oversimplification of groups of people relies on preconceived prejudice regarding these groups to provide narrative shortcuts that can be easily understood. Stereotypes are a popular technique employed by filmmakers representing disability. For example, people with disability are often stereotyped as villains or victims (Oliver, 1990). As Kriegal explains, 'the cripple is threat and recipient of compassion, both to be damned and pitied – and frequently to be damned as he is pitied' (Kriegal, 1987, p. 32). For Kriegal, the 'quintessential literary cripple' is both feared and pitied and there has been little variation in imagery.

Influenced by such critical analysis of disability as evil in literature, theorisation about the representation of disability in cinema has evolved from three main stereotypes identified by Paul Longmore in a 1985 article (republished in 1987 and again in 2003). Longmore argues that all representations of disability are influenced by the fundamentally negative stereotypes of criminality, adjustment and sexuality. He maintained a common stereotype saw people with disability as evil monsters who would – if they could – destroy the non-disabled. Longmore argued that, despite an abundance of on screen characters with disability, audiences screen them out due to a fear of disablement. Filmmakers use this fear of disablement to draw on a long history of visual and emotional cues associated with disability to communicate character information quickly and effectively to the audience. Longmore maintained that through repetition, on both film and television, characterisations of people with disability as criminals and sexual and social outcasts have a material effect on the position of people with disability in society.

The identification of disabling stereotypes is increasingly problematised in critical disability studies for limiting the discussion of disability representations and audience interpretations (Mallett, 2009). For example, Shakespeare (1999) argues that arguments regarding positive and negative stereotypes fail to grasp the complexity of representation, and Snyder and Mitchell (2006) caution against dividing the representation of disability into a positive and negative binary opposition due to shifting historical values. They note that what might appear positive to one generation may not to another. Arguments regarding positive and negative stereotypes also fail to take into account context, active audiences, and the ways people make meaning from a number of sources.

Cinema of Isolation

Martin Norden, who identified 10 cinematic stereotypes of disability, adds another dimension to the analysis of disability within cinematic narrative codes through the observation that characters with disability are isolated through both typical storylines and also the ways these storylines are imagined through the language of cinema:

> The phenomenon of isolation is reflected not only in the typical storylines of the films but also to a large extent in the ways filmmakers have visualised the characters interacting with their environments; they have used the basic tools of

their trade – framing, editing, sound, lighting, set design elements (e.g. fences, windows, staircase banisters) to suggest physical or symbolic separation of disabled characters from the rest of society. (Norden, 1994)

This isolation is evident in *Million Dollar Baby* when Maggie sustains a spinal cord injury and then loses a leg due to bed sores. Following her injury, Maggie is depicted only in medical settings, her body is handled by medical staff and equipment in every scene. The story is no longer Maggie's, it is now Frankie's emotional journey. Medium shots show Frankie's reactions to what is happening while Maggie is framed in wide shot to take in the medical paraphernalia around her or closer in profile. Despite being transferred to a rehabilitation centre and a large portion of the film being focused on her training, she is never shown participating in physiotherapy. Eddie 'Scrap Iron' Dupris' voice over narrates Maggie's predicament once she becomes disabled – the only time she is given voice herself is to tell her family to go away and ask Frankie to kill her.

Although Norden does not divide his analysis into specific genre types, the importance of genre is evident throughout his book as he alludes to the construction of disabled characters within particular genres such as the horror, film noir, western and melodrama and the tendency of specific genre types to be in and out of 'vogue' in Hollywood. Norden maintains that disability in the movies both reflects social values and works as a 'politically charged commodity that moviegoers are asking audiences to "buy"' (p. x). He encourages audiences to question how they are being positioned and what these images are selling them.

Body Genres

Snyder and Mitchell (2006) describe comedy, horror and melodrama as the foundational genres of film narratives and argue that disability is foundational to the ways audiences relate to these genres. Drawing on Linda Williams' argument that these three genres seek to invoke an emotional response from the audience, Snyder and Mitchell seek to contribute to a cultural investigation of disability in cinema by exploring the ways disability is used to elicit particular emotional responses such as disgust, pity and superiority (165). They argue that disability is as crucial to genre as gender in directing the narrative and the meaning made via audience identification.

For example, melodramas often make use of acquired impairments to invoke pity in the audience. Snyder and Mitchell explain that these narratives leverage audience concern about the fragility of their own bodies. Narratives usually conclude with body restoration and the negation of disability. Or, as in the case of *Million Dollar Baby*, the character with disability dies a merciful death.

Horrors by comparison, explore 'inborn monstrosity' to elicit feelings of disgust. In addition, characters may, as Longmore (1987) describes, seek to enact revenge. Freddy Kruger, the main character of the *Nightmare on Elm Street* cycle of horror films, is a clear example of this. With a burnt face and knives for fingers, Kruger is described in the film as 'the bastard son of a hundred maniacs'. He was conceived after a young girl was repeatedly raped while being held prisoner at a psychiatric hospital in the small American town of Springwood. After a turbulent childhood being moved around numerous foster homes, Kruger returns to Springwood and, disgusted by the picture-perfect image the town projects, goes on a murderous killing spree to enact revenge on the town that did not protect his mother nor himself. His actions were so evil that, when he was murdered by the townsfolk, dream demons in hell promised him eternal life in the world of dreams. And so Freddy began haunting the children of Elm Street in their dreams. Similarly, Jason of the *Halloween* films and Leatherface of *The Texas Chainsaw Massacre* are both constructed as mentally unstable murderous monsters whose physical impairments act as clear cinematic codes communicating their inherent evil.

Finally, comedies draw on faked impairment to elicit an emotional response of superiority while humiliation plays a key part in narrative resolution. Thomas Edison's 1898 short film *Fake Beggar* – which is often described as the first disability-themed film in Hollywood history – features faked impairment in its ridicule of disability. In the film, a beggar who pretends to be blind is caught out and comically chased by a policeman.

More recently, faked impairments have featured in the 'gross-out' cinema of the Farrelly brothers popular in the 1990s and early 2000s. Their break out hit *There's Something About Mary* is particularly notable for its use of disabled characters, including faked impairment. In addition to including a genuinely disabled character – Mary's brother Warren who operates as a 'defining other' against whom major character's redeeming features are measured – Tucker, one of the men vying for Mary's affections, pretends to have cerebral palsy in the hopes of seducing her. While the ruse does provide him greater access to Mary, she does not view him romantically. Other Farrelly brothers films such as *Dumb and Dumber*, *Me, Myself and Irene* and *Stuck on You* include characters with disability as sources of ridicule. The faked impairment continues to get quite an outing in these films through both major and minor characters. Whereas Snyder and Mitchell (2006) describe Farrelly brothers' films as hinging 'upon narrow ideas about unacceptable bodies that encourage freak-show-like titillation, as well as humor born of an all-too-easy superiority toward each character's bumbling incompetencies' (p. 191), Niall Richardson (2010) argues they 'might suggest the possibility of something quite transgressive but they always contain this threat within a very conventional narrative' (p. 191). Thus any transgression is quickly contained to reinforce a presumed non-disabled audience superiority.

Problem Bodies

In the introduction to their edited collection *The Problem Body*, Sally Chivers and Nicole Markotić maintain that, unlike other marginalised groups, disability is highly visible onscreen and, indeed, is vital to an ongoing cultural debate about the 'ideal norm of the human body' (p. 1). Rather than discuss *disability* per se, Chivers and Markotić invite a questioning of the *problem body* in cinema. 'Problem bodies' are broadly defined as – but not confined to – representations of disability, illness, ageing, obesity and other bodies which destabilise the ideal norm. Through a focus on the filmic projection of problem bodies, Chivers and Markotić seek to contribute to a post-Mulvey mode of film analysis that redirects 'the gaze' towards contemporary social issues. Rather than simply identify damaging stereotypes, they consider the way filmic narrative and mise-en-scène create the problem body.

The problem body enquiry that Chivers and Markotić recommend follows Snyder and Mitchell's cultural model and reveals the importance of considering genre and generic conventions when investigating disability in film. Although Snyder and Mitchell praise science fiction titles such as *Gattaca*, *Unbreakable* and the *X-Men* movies for their 'counter discursive forays' where disability becomes central to the plot rather than as a freak encounter, they do not explore science fiction in depth (p. 167).

Disability and Science Fiction

Science fiction cinema is a particularly rich field in which to observe changing social and political perspectives. The features of this genre have changed over time as a result of both technological and social changes. Advances in special effects have seen major changes to narrative pacing and audience expectation. Although most narratives are located in the future, present-day shifting social anxieties are explored in science fiction. For example, whereas films from the 1950s reflect a fear of invasion related to the Cold War, post-September 11 films display a fear of terrorism. Shifting gender roles can also be seen, as women do not take on leading roles in early science fiction cinema. Johnson Cheu (2002) notes that, although science fiction is preoccupied with medical intervention to cure human bodies of disabling impairments, disability continues to exist in these futuristic settings due to disabling social beliefs and expectations. Further, Kathryn Allan (2013) contends that these films problematise the utopian medicine as the ultimate cure argument and demand a consideration of contemporary socially imposed limitations. As Allan explains:

[Science fiction] takes the abnormal body, the novel form, and reimagines its usefulness. Instead of viewing bodily variation as deviancy, many SF texts reframe the disabled body not only as monstrous but also adaptive and subversive. … Since much SF takes up issues of technology, the notion of the body as tool becomes repositioned or reframed through the lens of disability studies. While SF undoubtedly recuperates stereotypical and biased views of the disabled body, the potential for reading – and imagining – alternative human bodies as transformative in the genre is worthy of sustained critical attention. (p. 8)

Science fiction's concern with the 'possible future of humanity' (Allan, 2013, p. 1) provides fertile source material for disability studies' aim of social inclusion. Science fiction interrogates questions of disability, ability, embodiment and identity, and offers disability a prominent position in popular culture. Allan observes that popular audiences gain the majority of their experiences with disability through science fiction representations which have long embraced monstrosity, deviance and deformity, and/or have used disabled characters to communicate a host of marginalised otherness. For Allan, disability has long been a concern of science fiction, from Mary Shelly's *Frankenstein* to the recent Hollywood blockbuster *Avatar*, and maintains that the genre offers an articulate critique of social anxieties.

Allan's explanation of science fiction as offering social critique and the opportunity for identification with a disabled embodiment despite reinforcing present-day stereotypes and prejudices positions science fiction as a producerly text. Disability studies reflect long-standing traditions of the science fiction genre as it explores the future possibilities of the human body in an environment constantly changed by humans. Both disability studies and science fiction are concerned with physical difference, body modification, environmental adaptation, medical research and notions of technological transcendence. Allan's observation that post-human utopias cannot obscure the reality that social disadvantage will continue to exist is of particular interest to disability analysis within science fiction.

Drawing on Müller, Klijn and Van Zoonen's (2012) argument that the most persistent representation of disability is the supercripple characterisation identified by a number of disability theorists, the next section offers a reading of the science fiction film *Gattaca* as perpetuating damaging stereotypes of disability, before later in the chapter taking up the notion that the film introduces social model critiques through the conventions of the cyberpunk subgenre of science fiction cinema.

Stereotypes of Disability in Gattaca: *Supercripple versus Own Worst and Only Enemy*[1]

In *Gattaca,* discrimination has advanced to the level of 'science'. Anne Finger (1998) finds parallels with the discrimination experienced by the 'de-gene-erates' of the film and actual people with disability. She goes on to identify that, while *Gattaca* is cautioning against a world where 'success is determined by science', its audience would largely consist of the so-called 'degenerates' of the film. Rather than leave the audience in the uncomfortable position of feeling discriminated against as degenerates, the film offers a disabled character recognisable by current standards who is ultimately shown to be weaker and lacking in desire to succeed. By comparison, the degenerate – with whom the audience is likely to identify – is depicted as refusing to accept socially imposed limitations and of rising above his predetermined position in life.

Colin Barnes (1992) compares two stereotypes of disability which he describes as the 'supercripple' and 'own worst and only enemy'. As I discussed in Chapter 3, the supercripple is the character with disability who *conquers* individual limitations and personal tragedy through a positive personal attitude, hard work and determination. While the supercripple advances a stiff upper lip approach to triumphing over adversary, it ignores the 'central point that disability is a social issue which cannot be addressed by misplaced sentimentality over individual impairments' (Barnes, 1992, p. 13). Barnes outlines the possible negative implications of these representations in terms of an individualisation of disability resulting in a denial of essential services such as the availability of braille and lip reading translations. He concludes that by 'focusing on a disabled individual's achievements such imagery encourages the view that disabled people have to overcompensate to be accepted into the community' (Barnes, 1992, p. 14).

Vincent is presented as a supercripple at several points throughout *Gattaca.* The film emphasises his drive to succeed 'despite' his genetic makeup. Throughout his life Vincent was tormented by his genetically superior brother Anton. As a youth, Vincent and Anton race in the ocean and Vincent becomes tangled in seaweed and loses the competition. However, later in the film, when the brothers re-enact this race, Vincent wins. When Anton asks how Vincent could have possibly won, and further risen to the heights in his career with the physical limitations he has, Vincent responds that he never saved any energy for the swim back to shore. In effect, Vincent was willing to give it his all – to die – to succeed.

---

1   Some material in this section has appeared in print before at Ellis, K. (2003). Reinforcing the Stigma – the Representation of Disability in Gattaca. *Australian Screen Education* (31), 111–14. Available through ATOM (http://www.metromagazine.com.au).

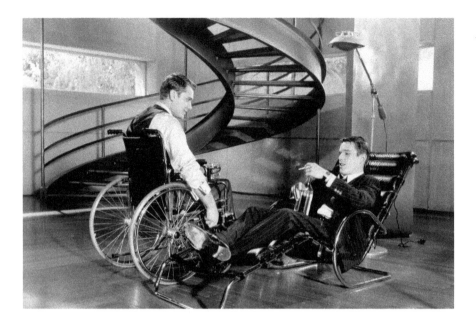

Figure 4.1   Jude Law as Jerome and Ethan Hawke as Vincent in *Gattaca*
Source: © Columbia Pictures courtesy of Photofest.

By comparison, the 'own worst and only enemy' stereotype is a straightforward opposite of the supercripple and portrays people with disability as 'self pitiers who could overcome their difficulties if they would stop feeling sorry for themselves, think positively and rise to "the challenge"' (Barnes, 1992, p. 14). Barnes again locates the origins of this stereotype in a medical or individual approach to disability which 'allows able-bodied society to reinterpret disabled people's legitimate anger over disablism as self-destructive bitterness arising out of their inability to accept the "limitations" of impairment' (p. 15). This construction, for Barnes (1992), neutralises any anger people with disability may express for a lack of essential services.

While Vincent refuses to accept the life expected of someone of his genetic makeup, Jerome embraces self-pity and becomes his 'own worst and only enemy'. He is stereotypically disabled – he has no friends, chain-smokes and drinks too much. The first image of Jerome ascribes to Norden's cinema of isolation – he wheels into an empty room looking defeated; he has resorted to selling his genes. Everything in the film looks high-tech except Jerome's wheelchair. The squeaking chair repositions disability as historical and non-existent in the future, yet the discrimination remains. Later scenes utilise the cinematic tools Norden referred to earlier such as a spiral staircase (see Figure 4.1) which works to separate Jerome in his wheelchair from able-bodied characters in the film. In a later scene, both Vincent and Jerome gaze at Gattaca. Vincent on crutches and Jerome in his wheelchair occupy the same 'disabled' position in that moment. However, as Vincent explains in voiceover, whereas he did not have the genes to get into Gattaca, Jerome did not have the desire.

Jerome has always shown signs of weakness – he came second when he was an athlete and he failed when he tried to kill himself, surviving as a paraplegic. He couldn't handle being the best, he couldn't pull it off, but Vincent can. Jerome is his own worst and only enemy – if Vincent can rise to the challenge, surely Jerome with his superior genes and privileged social position can. As Vincent realises his dream and travels into space, Jerome kills himself. As his body is engulfed in flames, the silver medal he wears around his neck turns gold – this is the first time Jerome is shown as winning.

Future Human Beings?

Recent science fiction displays a fascination with the human body as shaped by scientific, medical and information technologies and interventions. The scientific philosophy transhumanism posits that we are in an early phase of the technological evolution of the human body, and features in science fiction through artificial realities, limbs, cyborgs and amborgs (ambiguous human hybrids). Susan Schneider (2009) predicts that 'future human beings will be very unlike their present-day incarnation in both physical and mental respects', and may in fact resemble science fiction characters. She also predicts that people who do not embrace scientific enhancement to improve their 'basic capabilities' will appear 'intellectually disabled' (Schneider, 2009). They might also seem, as Vincent is in *Gattaca*, physically disabled because science and medicine demands an enhanced body.

Ramez Naam takes up this notion in *More Than Human: Embracing the Promise of Biological Enhancement* to argue we are in an early stage of human development and it will be possible to alter the body to enhance its capabilities. Throughout his book, Naam identifies numerous research projects attempting to find ways to cure disability and age related ailments that can be used to enhance human abilities in general (p. 5). For example, Naam explains that research into curing muscular dystrophy has produced super strong mice whose physicality surpasses that of unenhanced mice. Similarly, Naam observes that research into curing paralysis and amputation has seen monkeys implanted with electrodes able to move mechanical arms attached to their bodies. Research that allows people with vision impairment to see through connecting eyeglasses to electrodes in the visual parts of the brain could radically alter the way sighted people communicate. Naam explains that the scientists conducting these experiments have the common goal of '[healing] the sick and injured' (p. 6) but are also discovering ways to alter ourselves to 'benefit' society and improve our minds and bodies.

Naam argues that these advances in technology are debated by ethicists and politicians, with many emphasising the negatives of pursuing techniques to enhance human abilities. Naam takes the opposite position to bio-ethicists who argue that certain technological and medical interventions (such as the reproductive technologies explored in *Gattaca*) be banned outright. Curing people with disability of their impairments and the broader possibilities of altering everyone for optimum performance and communication is a theme that runs throughout Naam's book – a theme that is also interrogated in both science fiction cinema and critical disability studies.

Disability theorists such as Fiona Kumari Campbell (2009) critique the culture of an 'ethics of compulsory correction' (p. 96) that has emerged around technologies and surgeries to enhance quality of life for people with disability and the way in which they rely on ableism. Popular science fiction cinema also actively interrogates such predictions. For example, *Serenity* explores the use of technology to alter the human body for optimum work performance through the effects of such experiments on River and the inhabitants of the outer planet Miranda. One such example is when, in seeking to eradicate anger and aggression, the Alliance release a chemical through the air conditioning on Miranda. The result is that the majority of the population become so placid that they stop talking to each other or going to work; they basically give up breathing and die. The remaining one per cent, however, become even more aggressive. They become 'Reavers', a group of aggressive cannibal rapists who terrorise the outer galaxy and destroy all of Miranda. Similarly, in trying to create the perfect assassin in River, the Alliance destroy her emotional centre. Although *Serenity* is located in the imagined realm of science fiction, the film, along with disability studies broadly, clearly introduces important critiques about a possible future where humans are technologically 'enhanced'.

Naam (2012) does recognise that the enhancements he describes will not be available to everyone and argues we need to find a way to ensure they are. Thus, new forms of class related disability will be created in futuristic worlds, even if all impairments are cured (Johnson, 2002). With its focus on the workforce and loss of familial bonds, this issue is frequently debated within the cyberpunk subgenre of science fiction cinema.

Cyberpunk (Anxiety) to Post-cyberpunk (Acceptance)

In 1997 Nickianne Moody published an article entitled *Untapped Potential: The Representation of Disability/Special Ability in the Cyberpunk Workforce* which built on the foundations of the social model of disability to explore the representation of disability in cyberpunk literature and cinema. She argues that disabled and impaired characters occupy a different position within the cyberpunk genre where they become a 'visible and incidental part of the everyday cyberpunk world' (Moody, 1997, p. 102) as opposed to a narrative or cinematic prosthesis designed to elicit an emotional response from the audience.

This genre is characterised by an acceptance of a high-tech (cyber) near-future but a rejection of middle class values (punk). As Lawrence Person explains in *Notes Toward a Postcyberpunk Manifesto*:

> Classic cyberpunk characters were marginalized, alienated loners who lived on the edge of society in generally dystopic futures where daily life was impacted by rapid technological change, an ubiquitous datasphere of computerized information, and invasive modification of the human body. (Person, 1998)

Person's manifesto can be clearly seen in *Gattaca* as both Vincent and Jerome are alienated loners existing on the fringes of a dystopic future where daily life is dominated by technology and bodies are only valued if they have been genetically pre-planned. Thus cyberpunk recognises the dystopian future that over-reliance on technology could bring about.

Moody tracked the incidence of disabled characters appearing in this genre to demonstrate the way that everyone in cyberpunk is disabled by social expectations regarding work. She identifies the same three waves of social development that Finkelstein outlines in his three stages of disability development – agrarian society, the industrial revolution and the information age. While these phases are important to cyberpunk because, as a genre, it is preoccupied with work, a popular cultural studies concern with leisure is also prominent. Films belonging to this science fiction subgenre are set in a post-industrial future in which space-time relations have been altered and the dialectic between disability and impairment is resolved as long as people are working. Moody (1997) argues 'social integration is assured as long as [characters] are working, whether in the corporate marketplace or black economy' (p. 91). Knowledge and technology replace labour and capital as the 'central variables' of the economy. The cyberpunk future Moody and Person describe is a direct correlation to Finkelstein's third stage of disability where technological innovations foster greater inclusion of people with disability in the workforce. Finkelstein (1980) saw this inclusion as having a direct impact on institutions, practices and ideas. However, this conception of the future could produce new forms of disability, in the same way that the industrial revolution did.

Moody sees these news forms of disability being explored in cyberpunk through its dystopian vision of the new work environment. People lose familial bonds in deference to allegiance to 'corporations' who offer a sense of community belonging. In these worlds, the disabled emerge as a counter culture. For example, a disabled underground exists in *Gattaca* – it is revealed at the end of the film that several people have been helping Vincent succeed because they too belong to this underground by virtue of their own or their children's genetic makeup. For example Dr Lamar, who conducts genetic testing on Vincent's urine throughout the film, reveals he has known about Vincent's invalid status as he is about to launch into space. Lamar refers to his son, whose genetic makeup was 'not all that was promised', as a big fan. However, some characters, such as Vincent's brother Anton, side with the corporate order over their own familial bonds. Similarly, River and Simon's parents in *Serenity* disown their children to stay in the good graces of the Alliance and continue to live in the inner planetary system.

By comparison, Johnson Cheu (2002) interprets these science fiction films as being characterised by a medically-advanced futuristic setting preoccupied with curing disability. However, as Cheu explains, a rethinking of disability in terms of social stigma rather than medical affliction reveals that disability will not be eradicated or cured in the future. Instead, the social weight of disability will continue to be applied to other groups and people through class inequalities. Cheu identifies a class system operating in *Gattaca* where people with disability must either attempt to pass (Vincent), kill themselves if they can't (Jerome) or operate as a source of entertainment, as in the case of the concert pianist minor character referred to in the film as the 12-fingered man.

Moody (1997) attributes these medical interventions to corporations' goals to eradicate human frailty in order to optimise work performance. Such goals are problematised in *Serenity*. Although the Alliance (representative of Moody's 'corporation' and perhaps capitalism in general) has propagated a message that Reavers are 'men that went insane at the edge of space and became savage', they are the result of a failed Alliance experiment to eradicate undesirable human qualities. However, *Serenity* can also be seen to be exhibiting more optimism than other cyberpunk films such as *Gattaca*. Whereas Vincent flies into space as Jerome kills himself, *Serenity* ends with Simon and Kaylee making love and River serving as Mal's co-pilot.

Serenity thus progresses beyond cyberpunk cinema towards a genre that can be described as post-cyberpunk. Post-cyberpunk, although set in the same immersive world environments as cyberpunk, displays more optimism for the future. This sub subgenre of science fiction parallels our increasing reliance on computerised technology in both work and leisure. Post-cyberpunk features a different brand of characters who differ from the alienated loners of cyberpunk in the sense that they:

> ... are frequently integral members of society (i.e., they have jobs). They live in futures that are not necessarily dystopic (indeed, they are often suffused with an optimism that ranges from cautious to exuberant), but their everyday lives are

still impacted by rapid technological change and an omnipresent computerized infrastructure. (Person, 1998)

Similarly, Kimberly N. Rosenfeld (2010) notes a shift in public attitudes regarding the ways technology shapes our lives. She argues that, whereas cyberpunk films of the 1980s and 1990s exhibit anxiety and alienation, a new conception of the human–technology relationship is offered in contemporary films such as *Avatar* – 'Avatar's themes of hybridisation, fragmentation and hyperreality are not social liabilities rather, to a large extent, they can be read as transformative assets' (Rosenfeld, 2010). She compares the problem bodies of the cyborg human-machine in the *Terminator* films to the post-human problem body in *Avatar* to offer a framework for thinking about social critique in the context of 'mass-market appeal, impressive visuals, predictable characters, and surface-level storytelling'. Although she does not undertake a disability-informed critique, she observes the importance of Jake's physical impairments in what she describes as an investigation of 'today's political and social power and hegemonic ideology' (Rosenfeld, 2010).

Avatar: A Case Study

In the year 2154 the Earth is in the midst of an energy crisis and must acquire an energy mineral called 'unobtanium' for its survival in James Cameron's film *Avatar*. Unobtanium is in vast supply on the outer moon Pandora; however, Pandora's atmosphere is toxic to humans and the moon is populated by the unsympathetic Na'vi tribe. A colony of scientists and military have taken up residence on Pandora in the hopes of securing the unobtanium. Botanist Dr Grace Augustine has successfully developed the avatar program which allows human 'drivers' to link their consciousness to remote controlled humanoid-Na'vi bodies (avatars), enabling them to exist in the toxic air. She has also had some success initiating cultural bonds with the Na'vis. Jake Sully, a disabled marine, is sent to Pandora in lieu of his recently deceased twin brother who had been a scientist employed by the program. Jake, who becomes able-bodied once again inside his brother's Na'vi avatar, is tasked with infiltrating the tribe but finds his loyalties shift as he falls in love with the chief's daughter.

Slavoj Žižek offers a scathing critique of the film, focusing on the predictable characters and surface-level storytelling to argue:

It is easy to discover, beneath the politically correct themes (an honest white guy siding with ecologically sound aborigines against the "military-industrial complex" of the imperialist invaders), an array of brutal racist motifs: a paraplegic outcast from earth is good enough to get the hand of a beautiful local princess, and to help the natives win the decisive battle. The film teaches us that the only choice the aborigines have is to be saved by the human beings or to be destroyed by them. In other words, they can choose either to be the victim of imperialist reality, or to play their allotted role in the white man's fantasy. (Žižek, 2010)

Žižek's critique implicitly raises two points which would benefit from a critical disability analysis. Firstly, his argument that the film attempts to make a social and cultural critique while reinforcing existing inequalities guides my analysis of *Avatar* as a producerly text. Secondly, implicit in Žižek's critique, is the notion that a disabled man is inferior. Žižek interpretation thus rests on the observation Mitchell and Snyder (2000) take regarding disability being culturally positioned as the 'real limitation from which to escape' (p. 2). My producerly approach to *Avatar* acknowledges both the features of the film that have already been recognised by a number of critics as ableist, and further argues that the film also repositions disability as not inferior through its cultural critique of the 'military-industrial complex'.

Avatar – which grossed over US$2.78 billion worldwide at the box office and won 61 awards (of 73 nominations) including three Oscars – is a critically, commercially and philosophically significant film of recent years that features a disabled protagonist. Yet it has been almost universally slammed in the disability blogosphere and within academia for its representation of disability. Important critiques of the film have explored issues such as compulsory able-bodiedness, crip drag (or the hiring of non-disabled actors to portray disabled characters), stereotypical portrayals of disability, the disabling language used in the marketing of the film, the ableist ideology permeating the dialogue in the film itself and the medicalised approach to curing disability through Jake who is essentially a science experiment.

Disability as Counter Culture in Avatar

In this section I wish to approach a rereading of *Avatar* as offering critiques of disabling social environments. *Avatar* takes a post-cyberpunk approach to many of the debates of cyberpunk, particularly those that centre on corporate interests dominating people's lives, the scientifically enhanced human body, the demands of the workforce creating new forms of disability and the ways biotechnology and informatics are shifting human consciousness.

My reading is informed by Mitchell and Snyder's (2006) argument that the negative stereotype approach to analysis identifies plots that emphasise individual isolation and extracts them from their social context, and Mallet's (2009) observation that a focus on stereotypes reproduces the same types of readings of disability. The remainder of the chapter explores three aspects of the representation of disability in *Avatar*. Firstly, the intriguing paradox that, while Jake is socially disabled throughout the entire film, he continues to exhibit masculine identity markers. Indeed, the high-tech future in which *Avatar* is set allows a disabled man to take on the leading role. Secondly, the avatar could be seen as prosthesis or mobility aid like a wheelchair – the fact that Jake chooses to stay within his avatar rather than receive medical treatment by aligning with the military problematises a reading of compulsory able-bodiedness. This is especially true given everyone's reliance on prostheses throughout the film. Finally, disability as counter culture is explored through the rejection of the military and corporation.

A Failed Marine?

Jake is disabled and rejected by the world he lives in after serving in a war which caused his impairment. It is revealed that Jake cannot afford a cure which, by all accounts, is readily available. He uses a small manual wheelchair (see Figure 4.2) that is arguably out-of-date by today's standards, perhaps because cures are available to those who can afford them and thus technological progress regarding mobility aids is not invested in. Just as in *Gattaca*, people with disability are therefore considered to be an underclass. Jake describes his motivations for going to Pandora in terms of viewing it as 'just another hell hole'.

In her review of the film for *Feminists with Disability for a Way Forward*, Ouyang Dan argues that, while it would be easy to write the film off as ableist, the narrative introduces some important critiques regarding the way people with disability are treated:

> This is a society that hasn't learned how to accept a person outside of the standard, and doesn't yet know how to accept them into their perfect world. Society doesn't know what to do with a Jake Sully because it doesn't want to … and why should it? It will just cast him off and get more fresh, able bodies to replace him. He isn't their problem any more, right? (Dan, 2010)

It can therefore be argued that, although disability has been medically eradicated in the fictional world of *Avatar*, social disadvantage continues to exist for those who cannot afford to pay for a cure. These people are disregarded and easily replaced by more able bodies. In comparison to life on Earth, where nature and humanity are ignored, the Na'vis approach all living things as interconnected. They seek to look inside one another to really know a person. Thus, while their physical bodies are the image of perfection, it is what's inside that counts. They express positive feelings about meeting someone by saying 'I see you'. The phrase is both a phatic form of communication and a cornerstone of Na'vi philosophy. If the Na'vis do indeed 'see' Jake, they know of his impairment.

The storyline of *Avatar* has been accused of replicating racist narratives whereby the colonial white hero rescues the natives in a similar vein to *Dances With Wolves* (Žižek, 2010). However, as a disabled man, and member of the underclass, Jake would be rejected by colonial power. In fact the avatar that 'liberates' him from his impaired body is not even his. He did not go to Pandora to become able-bodied, he went to work. It was not the promise of 'compulsory correction' that convinced him to go, it was the promise of 'good money'.

Jake occupies several disability positions and subjectivities throughout the film – he is disabled by every group he seeks to align with. Firstly, his physical impairment prevents him from being a marine. Despite this, Jake continues to view himself as a marine, believing he still has the attitude and could pass any test. When Jake arrives on Pandora along with other military personnel, the guards already there refer to the group as 'fresh meat' and Jake as 'meals on wheels'. Further, despite his background as a marine, his lack of scientific training see the scientists subjugate him for his perceived lack of intellect – he is both told not to say anything and to 'try to use big words'. Jake is shown to have no power. Much of his worth bound up in his body which Jake literally sacrificed for his country, yet they will not provide him with what appears to be basic medical care. Finally, the Na'vis recognise him as an avatar or 'dreamwalker' and describe him as being 'like a baby, making noise, don't know what to do'. He must learn their ways and undergo tests in order to be accepted.

By the end of the film, however, Jake has become the physical and psychological superior in each of these groups. If, as Dr Patel says in the film, 'good science is good observation', Jake has been able to observe the Na'vi like no one before him, even Dr Grace Augustine who literally 'wrote the book'. He defeats Colonel Quaritch and all of his hyper-masculine men by riding a toruk, a giant predatory animal native to Pandora. Jake is only the sixth Na'vi to conquer a toruk, making him a Na'vi hero. As Leigha McReynolds explains, Jake troubles the disability–ability binary:

> Because the Na'vi understanding of embodiment is so radically different from the human, Jake succeeds in part because of his experience with disability. As a paraplegic, Jake is familiar with the prosthetic through the use of a wheelchair. His transition from able-bodied to disabled already modified his understanding and practice of embodiment. It is possible that Jake's immediate facility with the avatar – a high tech biological prosthesis – can be attributed to this lived experience. (McReynolds, 2013, pp. 121–2)

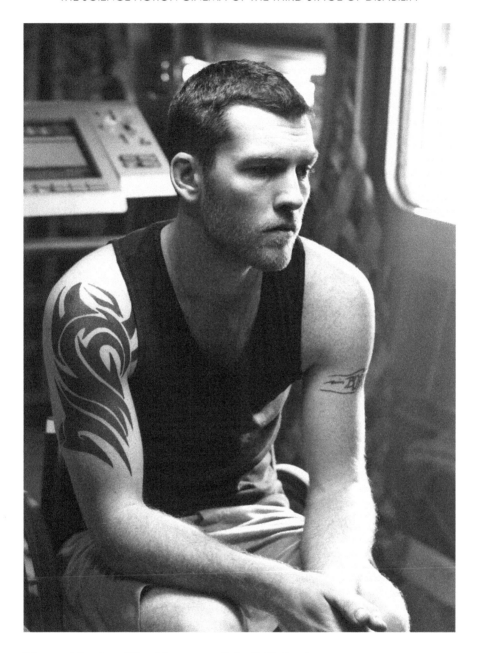

Figure 4.2 Sam Worthington as Jake Sully in *Avatar*

Source: © Twentieth Century-Fox Film Corporation courtesy of Photofest.

Prosthesis

McReynolds argues that the prosthesis in science fiction invites a new understanding of what is currently considered a disabled body. There is a scene within *Avatar* where Jake, having reclaimed an able body through his Na'vi avatar, runs, skips and wiggles his toes in the sand. The scene has both been criticised for perpetuating compulsory able-bodiedness (Palmer, 2011), and described as a realistic representation of what a person would do if they were suddenly to become able-bodied again (Dan, 2010). However, Jake has not just become able-bodied, he has become an amborg, an 'ambiguous hybrid' creature who is suddenly 4 metres tall and connected to all living things around him. As an amborg, however, Jake remains a 'problem body', although not necessarily disabled, except arguably by the Na'vis who differentiate him as a dreamwalker via his scent.

If a prosthesis can be defined something which 'allow[s] a body to function in an environment for which it is otherwise unequipped' (McReynolds, 2013, p. 115), then the Na'vi avatar body can be perceived as a another prosthesis, like the wheelchair, that allows Jake to exist in nature. Ultimately, Jake becomes an artificial human. The film questions the boundaries of what is human in an environment where capitalist values count for nothing. Even Grace, who is not disabled, feels her physical inferiority when she returns to her body after operating her avatar, referring to it as an 'old sack of bones'.

Drawing on Norden's cinema of isolation, Jake is not actually framed to suggest physical or symbolic isolation in terms of his masculinity. The scene where he discusses aligning with the military with Colonel Quaritch clearly illustrates this. Quaritch and Jake are always framed on an equal level and Quaritch takes great pains to align with Jake's sense of masculinity against the scientists who he describes as 'limp dick' and 'pukes'. The scene begins with Quaritch bench pressing, thereby working on strengthening his upper body as Jake uses his upper body to wheel into the room. The two then move to Quaritch's amplified mobility platform (AMP), a 4-metre tall, 2-metre wide robotic suit (another prosthesis) the military use to traverse Pandora, as they discuss Jake providing intelligence regarding how to force the Na'vis into submission. Jake sits on a platform at equal height. The only point in the interaction where Jake is framed as 'beneath' Quaritch is when Quaritch offers him his legs back, a prospect Jake ultimately rejects by the film's conclusion.

Rejection of Cure/Military/Corporation/Those who Disable

Jake's embrace of the Na'vi culture can equally be seen as a rejection of corporate disciplining regimes and an embrace of a disability counter culture. The Na'vi do not work and in fact refuse to bring in money for the corporation. They do not want to trade their ancestors' voices in the home tree for 'light beer and blue jeans'. In order for humans to exist alongside the Na'vi they must 'abandon their capitalist values and reinvent themselves to cohabitate respectfully and harmoniously with their environment and each other' (Rosenfeld, 2010).

Just as Jake realises he is having trouble differentiating reality (being a disabled former marine) from dream (living as a Na'vi in his avatar), Quaritch informs him that he has organised for Jake to rotate home where medical treatment for him to receive his 'real legs' back has been approved. Jake declines the offer, stating he wants to finish what he started. He is about to participate in the final ceremony that will 'make [him] a man' in the Na'vi culture.

In *Contours of Ableism*, Fiona Kumari Campbell (2009) questions whether a 'new relation between nature and culture' is emerging or if we are simply witnessing 'a new configuration of ableist relations based on intrinsic human-technological relation' (p. 45). *Avatar* asks the same question. As discussed, throughout the film everyone relies on prosthesis or cyborg or amborg support to exist in the world of Pandora. The military, scientists and corporate structure all make use of exopacks, a lightweight breathing apparatus to exist in the toxic air. The military become killing machines through their use of AMPs in which human bodies literally become fused with machines. The scientists, of course, make use of avatars and the Na'vis use the fibreoptic-like cables at the tip of their braids to fuse with flying banshees and dragons.

Further, the bond between the animals and Na'vi is quasi-telepathic; they communicate with their minds. The physical connection, and therefore body, is the conduit, the cable connecting the Na'vi to everything around them. Despite their physicality, it is what is inside a person's heart that matters. Jake, who earlier in the film described himself as having never lost the attitude of a marine although now unable to fight in combat, is able to capture the interest of the Na'vis who decide to observe him rather than kill him because he is the first warrior dreamwalker they have come across.

Conclusion

The majority of social model critiques of the representation of disability in cinema have proceeded from a social-realist perspective and taken literal interpretations of stereotypes/archetypes of disability represented in film. While cultural disability studies have identified the importance of disability to narrative discourse, few have embraced social critiques explored within the films themselves. Using science fiction cinema, this chapter approaches an intersection of both the social and cultural models of disability to explore the important disability debates taking place within this popular genre that has mass appeal.

As we proceed further into the third stage of disability outlined by Vic Finkelstein, it is possible more people will become disabled by new work demands placed on people and body modifications that may be out of reach for the majority of people. As such, science fiction is an important genre to explore with regards to the debates around disability in society. Within the broader science fiction genre, cyberpunk as a subgenre emerging during the 1980s takes up the critiques of the social model while introducing a further critique of the information age itself – that in the workforce of the future everyone is potentially disabled. As the anxiety around the human-machine relationship began dissipating during the 2010s, optimism has infused science fiction such as *Avatar*. While cyberpunk cinema such as *Gattaca* encourages us to think beyond the liberatory potential of the information age introduced by the social model, post-cyberpunk such as *Avatar* introduces optimism around technology while critiquing the disabling impact of corporate values – another key concern of the social model.

Chapter 5
Among the Leading Characters on Television

In 1992 Jack Nachbar and Kevin Lause argued that analysing unsuccessful popular culture offers insight into what is *not* within a cultural mindset at a particular moment in time. Drawing on the televisual dramatic mystery genre as 'one of the most consistently popular forms', they comment that the format reinforces popular cultural values regarding both family and the belief that justice will triumph even when the law fails (Nachbar and Lause, 1992, pp. 33–4). *Twin Peaks*, a technically accomplished mystery drama produced in 1990–91, challenged these assumptions; a strategy Nachbar and Lause argue resulted in its ratings failure:

> *Twin Peaks* challenged American beliefs in the simplicity and inherent decency of small town rural life (Twin Peaks, U.S.A. was a cesspool of violence, dangerous sex, and unexplained phenomena in the woods), the fundamentally supportive and protective character of the nuclear family, and the assurance that justice will triumph through the courageous fortitude of a righteous individual even when the law has failed (investigator Dale Cooper never solved anything and ended up being possessed by the very evil forces he was attempting to destroy). The failure of *Twin Peaks* suggests that these values still have a powerful hold on the American consciousness, and the fact that successful contemporary examples of the form *uphold* these same beliefs is even more evidence of such a conclusion. (Nachbar and Lause, 1992, p. 14)

Twin Peaks is an interesting example to make this point, not least because, despite not being listed in the top 50 programs of either season in its 2-year run, it amassed a dedicated and vocal cult following and arguably represents the fracture of the mass television audience into smaller niches. This audience fracture has been crucial in changing the way disability in represented on television.

TV reviewer Alan Sepinwall argues in his acclaimed self-published book *The Revolution Was Televised: The Cops, Crooks, Slingers and Slayers who Changed TV Drama Forever* that the recent diversification of television content pioneered a new type of storytelling and led to a revolution on our screens – an environment where television could be taken seriously. He identifies a number of television shows including, among others, *The Sopranos*, *Lost*, *Friday Night Lights* and *Breaking Bad* as 'game changers' in the television landscape. These programs, through a reckless mix of abandon and regret for past mistakes, targeted smaller and more diverse audiences. They took risks, they challenged cultural assumptions regarding family and law and justice. Significantly, these shows also included characters with disability or drew on disability themes.

Following Fiske's argument that television reflects rather than creates social change (Fiske, 1987, 2006, 1989, 2010), this chapter considers new types of representations that have emerged since the major theorisations of disability and television that occurred during the 1980s and 1990s through two indicative television texts – *Friday Night Lights* and *Push Girls*. These shows reveal that a struggle does exist for greater social inclusion and that gains have been made through the changing social position of disability.

The chapter begins with a general discussion of the specificity of television as a medium before moving on to outline prior research into television from a disability perspective. The chapter proceeds from Rosemarie Garland-Thomson's (2007) argument that community and sexuality can structure a positive story of disability by positioning characters' experiences as possible *because of* rather than *in spite of* their impairments. I begin with a reading of the US television series *Friday Night Lights*, in which the character Jason Street engages in the typical storylines of the high school drama while revealing both the effects of physical impairment and a disabling social world. What is notable about *Friday Night Lights* is the manner in which the program represents disability as the relationship between Jason's body, mind, self, society, and an environment that excludes him. The chapter then turns to how community and sexuality are debated in and around television entertainment using Season 1 of the reality TV series *Push Girls*. I consider the importance of both fan and antifan discussion of the issues around disability introduced in this series.

Television as Popular Culture, Art, Industry and Academic Discipline: From Mass Audiences to Niche Markets

In the previous chapter, I discussed the way cinema relies on specific narrative codes to communicate ideas about disability. A significant proportion of disability-informed research into disability and television proceeds from insights obtained through film analysis. However, it is important also to consider the specificity of television – namely what makes television television.

Television is characterised by a 'dialectic ... between art and industry, innovation and imitation, originality and repetition' (Gray, 2008, p. 19). As a form of popular culture, television holds much potential for an examination of disability. As Sepinwall observes, television can draw viewers in and make them care about what happens to the characters over a long period of time:

> It could tell very long stories. It could allow characters to grow over extended periods of time. And by coming into my home rather than making me go to it, it could forge a more intimate bond with me. (Sepinwall, 2012, p. 2)

This 'care factor' holds great potential for depictions of disability. Characters can be shown as developing and growing, as coming to terms with how to live with an acquired disability like Jason Street on *Friday Night Lights* or like Walt Jnr on *Breaking Bad* – the disability is just part of who they are and is not necessarily emphasised. Scott Porter, the actor portraying disabled character Jason Street on *Friday Night Lights*, describes the television serial format as integral to allowing a character with disability to grow in a way that cannot be achieved by the movie format:

> I've always said, with Jason, if a character gets this severely injured in a movie, they're done. But if you injure someone this severely on television, their journey is just beginning. (Porter cited on Coach G, 2007)

Broadcast television emerged in the 1950s, with most countries offering only three channels until the 1970s (Gray, 2008). A strategy of nation-building and family togetherness was adopted as networks targeted broad audiences (Katz, 2009) rather than smaller niche audiences as is more common today. A generalised experience was represented onscreen which, according to John Hartley (2010), *represented everyone* but allowed *no one* to speak for themselves (p. 119). And, thus, particular types of characters emerged through the lack of diversity. Specifically, because television is in the business of making money, formats and genres known to attract audiences are repeated in the hopes of replicating profits. As Nachbar and Lause (1992) discuss, dramatic mysteries bring in big audiences when they reinforce American values regarding the nuclear family and the fortitude of law enforcement and legal justice. While they note *Twin Peaks* did not succeed because it questioned these very values, the recent successes of programs like *Breaking Bad*, *Weeds* and *The Sopranos* suggest television has diversified since the initial broadcast era.

Significantly, for Gray (2008), television entertainment offers a 'massive cultural database and vocabulary we can access to discuss society – what it is, what it could be, and what we wish it was not' (p. 63). While television representations have been dissected from a number of perspectives to reveal the limited social roles available via this medium, recent insights in television studies note the importance of converging media platforms and the intersecting relationship between television and the online audience. Theorists recommend that we should pay as much attention to the online audience as we have previously paid to representations on television (Hartley, 2008). Perhaps where people with disability have been subject to distorted representations on television, online discussion could offer a form of rehabilitation where fans and antifans use television entertainment as an opportunity to discuss what society is and what it could be, and together narratise the society they actually want. Television and popular culture have changed since their early days – they now exist within an increasingly participatory environment where individuals cross international borders and attempt to influence the producers of popular culture while producing popular culture themselves.

Research into Disability on TV

The media – and television in particular – is consistently criticised for its representation of disability. Critiques concentrate on underrepresentation, negative stereotypes and inaccurate portrayals of normalisation (Müller, Klijn, and Van Zoonen, 2012). As Zhang and Haller (2013) observe, disability media studies has been dominated by content analysis for the last 30 years, with studies focusing on revealing 'problematic media representations of people with disabilities and their issues' (p. 321). For example, Guy Cumberbatch and Ralph Negrine's 6-week study in 1988 highlighted stereotypes and inconsistencies of disability on British prime-time television. They posited that, in order for social change to occur, people with disability needed to become 'among the leading characters' on television (Cumberbatch and Negrine, 1992, p. 140).

During the 1990s this type of research was replicated by other theorists who sought to build a more political framework into the analysis. For example, Colin Barnes (1992) conducted a content analysis using the social model of disability as the basis for identifying 'misrepresentation' of disability on television. For Barnes, the misrepresentation of disability on television was visible in 11 durable and overlapping stereotypes which he lists as pitiable and pathetic; object of violence; sinister and evil; atmosphere or curiosity; supercripple; object of ridicule; own worst and only enemy; burden; sexually abnormal; unable to participate in the community; and normal. He also provides a list of 'appropriate' contexts in which to represent disability, including avoiding associations with evil, charity, comedy, voyeurism and sensationalism. For Barnes, an interrogation of the discrimination experienced by people with disabilities is one of the only acceptable ways in which to represent disability on television. Like Longmore (discussed in the previous chapter) and Cumberbatch and Negrine, Barnes argued that the media teaches society about disability, and repetition of stereotypical portrayals perpetuates the values of 'less enlightened times' (Barnes, 1997, p. 5).

However, the social model that Barnes enthusiastically embraces has been questioned for its inability to speak for all people with disability. In addition, there have been a number of significant disability-specific social gains in the intervening years. For example, disability legislation was introduced in most Western societies during the 1990s, and the argument that disability is a central cultural identity and organising axis of power regarding status, wealth, gender, identity, bodies, life and death (Duncan, Goggin, and Newell, 2005) has more recently emerged as an important subfield within media studies. Social model and civil rights disability movements have challenged common sense assumptions about disability and revealed the socially created origins of disablement.

Nevertheless, content analysis has remained a favoured mode of research within disability studies, and other theorists have made similar arguments regarding the potential television represents regarding changing public attitudes about disability. For example, Saito and Ishiyama (2005) analysed the representation of disability on prime-time Japanese television between 1993 and 2002 and similarly found people with disabilities were underrepresented. They suggested that increasing the number of main characters with disabilities on prime-time television would change social attitudes and increase employment prospects for people with disabilities. While the presence of disabilities continues to dominate crime drama (Ellis and Goggin, 2015), factual programming and films (as we saw in Chapter 3), people with disabilities are also emerging as leading characters in other genres and formats and, importantly, in prime-time roles.

In addition to these changes in legislation, social standing and academic interest, there *are* leading characters with disabilities on television and narratives do reflect a degree of social change. Between 2010 and 2013 the US-based Gay and Lesbian Alliance Against Defamation (GLAAD) have included disability in their investigation of representations of diversity on television. In 2010, the number of series regular characters with a disability was six, dropping to four the following year. Then in 2013 the number rose to the still miniscule figure of eight (GLAAD, 2010; GLAAD (Gay and Lesbian Alliance Against Defamation), 2012, 2013) The GLAAD note that reality television programming which does not release participant information early enough to be included in the study represents some of the most diverse representation on television. Although their focus is on gay and lesbian people, reality television also holds great potential for the representation of disability (Müller et al., 2012).

Jonathan Gray notes that content analysis – the focus on the percentage of characters of a particular minority relative to the wider population lacks nuance. He explains that considering depictions as opposed to proportionality (Gray, 2008, p. 109) offers greater insight into a cultural mindset. *Parenthood*, a drama that features in GLAAD's list for the past 3 years, illustrates the importance of Gray's argument. While Max Braverman, a young boy with Asperger's on *Parenthood*, represents only one character with a disability on prime-time television, the narratives surrounding Max offer important insights into the experience of disability:

> The Asperger's storyline follows the family's journey to accept Max's diagnosis and help him progress, all while dealing with their own emotions. The show's heavy focus on life with a developmental disability is believed to be a first and so far audiences both with and without ties to autism seem to be responding. "While not all parents are dealing with autism or Asperger's, what I do find is all parents are dealing with something with their kids", says Jason Katims, the show's creator who himself has a son on the autism spectrum. (Diament, 2010)

Despite the traditional absence of series regular characters with disability, audiences of people with disability have long noticed their presence on screen in stereotypical roles (Ross, 1997, p. 669). Ross' study of audiences was an attempt to counter the emphasis on content analysis within disability studies. She proceeded from the perspective that disability is absent on screen; however, the participants with disability in her study focused on stereotypes of people with disability as criminals or outcasts, especially within soap operas. The participants saw these images as contributing to their social marginalisation (Ross, 1997, p. 669).

Alison Wilde's 2004 investigation found similar tendencies but also noted that audiences with disabilities tended to identify more with non-disabled television characters rather than their onscreen disabled counterparts. Kama's (2004) investigation of Israeli audiences also found that stereotypes of inspiration and tragedy dominated. Other research shows that people with disabilities tend to embrace gender divisions when it comes to program selection, for example men watch sports and women watch soaps despite being treated as *genderless* in other aspects of their lives (Gutierrez and Martorell, 2011).

In his 1992 investigation of disability on television, Colin Barnes – who was critical of Cumberbatch and Negrine (1992) for their lack of social model political conviction – argued that people with disabilities needed to be recruited as workers at all levels of the media industries, that characters with disabilities be portrayed only by actors with disabilities, and that the media seek advice from actual people with disabilities. This advice is now being given freely by audience members who engage with television plot lines on online forums and in blogs. Analysis of this online discourse regarding disability is providing disability researchers new insight to the ways audiences interpret televisual representations of disability.

For example, in their analysis of blogger discourse surrounding the 2007 remake of the *Bionic Woman*, Quinlan and Bates (2009) argue that the program uniquely brings together representations of gender, disability and cyborgs. They identify these themes being discussed in the blogger discourses surrounding the show in ways that both reinforce and resist disabling social values. Significantly, they also note a shift in social values when comparing the 1970s *Bionic Woman* to the 2007 remake, 'The two versions reflect the times in America when they aired' (p. 51).

As Quinlan and Bates notes, big drama television productions such as the *Bionic Woman* offer a uniquely televisual opportunity to consider disability and its relationship with changing social values. Another example is the US television series *Friday Night Lights*, which introduces important critiques around disability inclusion.

Drama: *Friday Night Lights* and Shape Structures Story[1]

Friday Night Lights is set in the fictional town of Dillon, Texas where the community is defined by high school football. The series begins with the high hopes for the Dillon High School Panthers now that they have secured promising new coach Eric Taylor. The team is made up of a group of promising young athletes but, most significantly, the quarterback Jason Street has been ranked the best quarterback not only in Texas but nationally. The aspirations of this working-class town rest on Jason's shoulders as he takes to the field in the first football game of the season. When Jason takes a bad tackle and is seriously injured, the entire community stops as they watch him lying motionless on the oval. As the spectators whisper to each other, the commentators lament the seriousness of the situation and medics hypothesise that it is a spinal cord injury. Jason is rushed to the hospital where it is discovered he has indeed sustained such an injury. Jason's injury and subsequent disablement, both physical and social, drive *Friday Night Lights* for three seasons.

Friday Night Lights creator Peter Berg envisioned television as a medium that would allow the story – a small community bonded through high school football which had previously been released as a book and movie – to 'go deeper' into complex issues. The disablement of the town's star quarterback was written into the television iteration serving as a 'clear dramatic climax' (Sepinwall, 2012, p. 276). Berg's comments reflect a clearly manipulative use of disability, a strategy often employed by television producers and, just as often, criticised by disability theorists and popular culture bloggers. However, a consideration of Jason's character progression reveals a number of important disability representations.

---

1 Some material in this section has appeared in print before at Ellis, K. (2012). 'Because of rather than in spite of: "Friday Night Lights" important cultural work of intersecting disability and masculinity'. *Interactive Media* issue 8 http://nass.murdoch. edu.au/nass_im_ejournal.htm.

Community and a More Political View of Disability

The high school quarterback at once represents community, teenage sexuality and masculinity in and beyond American popular culture. By featuring an elite high school quarterback becoming disabled, *Friday Night Lights* began with a storyline that subverts this cultural paradigm. *Friday Night Lights* is unique because people with disability are usually excluded from narratives of community and sexuality (Garland-Thomson, 2007). Just as Gray encourages analysis of depictions as opposed to proportions grounded in content analysis, Garland-Thomson encourages a recognition of the recasting of traditional disability plots through stories possible *because of* rather than *in spite of* disability. She identifies sexuality and community as two instances where narratives do the cultural work of re-engaging disability. For example, as I discuss in Chapter 7, in the acclaimed documentary *Murderball*, the presence of the wheelchair does not signal a loss of masculinity, rather it offers access to a hyper-masculine world – you must be disabled to play quad rugby.

A similar narrative trajectory, albeit within the confines of a television drama, takes place with Jason Street on *Friday Night Lights*. The program rewrites the usual narrative of disability in relation to community, sexuality and gender as Jason maintains everyday life without denying the significance of his disability. Although disabled, Jason participates in the typical storylines of a teenaged character in a soap opera. His experience with disability provides the opportunity to consider a number of political issues within the same narrative such as inaccessibility, access to rehabilitation, housing and employment, prejudice, and the process of adjusting to a new life with a disability.

Narrative dramas introducing characters who become disabled often depict these characters as hopeless and socially dead. These dramas rarely depict a rehabilitation process that demonstrates the alternative ways people with disability can participate in the community. For example, Sean, a character with a disability introduced for one episode (episode 18, series 1 'Laryngitis') in the popular television series *Glee*, has a very similar story to Jason – both characters have sustained spinal cord injuries during a high school football game. However, while Sean is always in bed, Jason is shown not only participating in physiotherapy on a rehabilitation process, but is also portrayed in his everyday life using modified utensils such as a fork to cut his own food or a straw to drink.

Initially Jason struggles to find his place in the community and his old friends have difficulty relating to him because he will never walk or play football again. When the team visit him in hospital they are visibly uncomfortable. Later, when Jason is wheeled out onto the football field before a Panthers game, the silence of the shocked crowd is in stark contrast to the exuberant cheers Jason received as the star quarterback in the first episode. They applaud only when instructed to do so. Herc, who attends rehab with Jason, takes issue with

Jason being treated as a mascot and begins introducing him to a more political view of disability – one that will eventually give Jason an identity and purpose. Significantly, Jason is unable to re-enter the football community until he accepts that he has become disabled and starts identifying with people with disabilities.

While the story generated from Jason's traumatic injury provides the dramatic impetus for *Friday Night Lights*, his and others' characters develop constantly throughout this show. Jason's accident is, without doubt, extremely traumatic for him and those close to him. In the pilot, Coach Taylor describes the accident as a test and a reminder that everyone is vulnerable. Despite the obvious similarities to 'inspirational' stories common on soaps and other broadcast programs, *Friday Night Lights* follows the trajectory Garland-Thomson (2007) sees as structuring a positive story – community and sexuality in a masculine context.

Masculinity and Sexuality

Jason plays a fairly traditional sick role until 'Crossing the Line' (episode 8, series 1). By this time in the story Jason has begun to settle into his new life through sport and community. However, after discovering his girlfriend (Lyla) and best friend (Tim Riggins) have been having an affair, he initiates a fight with Riggins. This is an overt signal towards Jason reclaiming his sexuality and masculinity. Herc – older, tougher and more politically aware than Jason – is integral to this journey. He urges Jason to stop taking 'crumbs'. For example, he is horrified that Jason continues to be in a relationship with Lyla despite her infidelities and tells Jason that by keeping the girlfriend he had when he could walk he avoids the reality that he is one of them – disabled.

Herc introduces Jason to the extremely masculine sport of wheelchair rugby – murderball. Here, *Friday Night Lights* relies on a narrative structure that emphasises real life situations as opposed to contrived situations, for example Jason is not immediately successful when trying out for the team as team managers believe he is not 'comfortable in [his] chair yet'. They encourage him to adjust to his new identity as a person with a disability. Despite this rejection, his involvement in an extremely masculine sport that requires athletes to be disabled allows Jason a way to reconnect with football – the sport that defined him – in a new way. He begins mentoring the Panther's struggling new quarterback Matt Saracen and reconciles with Riggins. While television often focuses on stories of superhuman achievement, *Friday Night Lights* recognises the necessity of a period of readjustment. An example of this is when Jason moves further towards a disability community by watching videos of murderball games and getting out of bed at 6am to train in the episode entitled 'Nevermind' (1.11).

The camera angles deployed in *Friday Night Lights* are also of interest. The producers utilise a political and innovative filming style, for example when Jason does break up with Lyla, the camera is at his chair height during their argument.

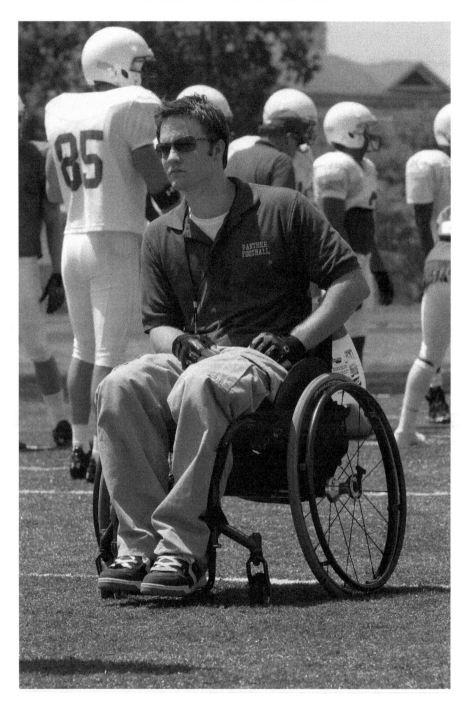

Figure 5.1   Scott Porter as Jason Street in *Friday Night Lights*, 2006

Source: © NBC via Getty Images.

A similar camera technique was used in the 1978 Vietnam War film *Coming Home* to avoid a semiotic connection with powerlessness (Norden, 1994). It was believed that putting the camera at the same height of their wheelchairs gave the men in *Coming Home* agency in the shot. Whereas most films 'looked down' on characters who used wheelchairs, Haskell Wexler the cinematographer for *Coming Home* wanted to depict his characters as masculine and empowered. *Friday Night Lights* uses and inverts the same technique throughout the following episodes as the camera remains at Jason's chair height, giving him prominence in the frame, except when the narrative is dealing with instances of social disablement. In those scenes, the camera looks down on Jason to reflect his social disempowerment. The semiotic connection with powerlessness is seen in episode 19 'Ch-Ch-Ch-Ch-Changes' when Jason is refused the sale of beer for being underage. The irony is highlighted when Riggins, the next customer and exactly the same age, has no problems buying them both alcohol simply because he is a football player and small town hero.

Sexuality, the second narrative current identified by Garland-Thomson (2007), is also emphasised in this episode. Where previously in 'Crossing the Line' Jason initiates an argument with Lyla instead of having sex with her, in 'Nevermind' Jason admits he can't feel anything and is nervous at the prospect of having sex. While this motivates Lyla to track down an instructional video, Jason asks Herc for advice, who tells him that he will need to relearn everything just as a newborn baby would. He needs to figure out what works for him because everything is different now. Jason's experience with disability shapes several subplots in the context of teenaged sexuality. In later episodes he has both one-night stands and longer-term girlfriends, including an engagement which he ended. One of his sexual encounters results in the birth of a child and – in the tradition of soap opera – marriage.

Following a period of adjustment, Jason achieves self-assurance through involvement with the disability community and begins to enter sexual relationships with confidence. He also continues to be heavily involved in the sporting community, both football and quad rugby. Jason and his family and friends experience difficulties related to both the physical effects of his impairment and the social stigmas and power imbalances that surround them. This characterisation acknowledges disability – both as socially created and limitations that relate to embodiment.

Having an ongoing series regular character with disability allowed *Friday Night Lights* to introduce a number of concerns relevant to the disability experience, including the issues of community and sexuality discussed above, depression surrounding a changing embodiment, a search for a cure, retrofitting access, finding employment, appropriate housing and dealing with a disabling society. Some of these narratives would be considered positive, others negative, and certainly Jason is only one character on one television show. As indicative of people with disability, Jason may represent an unattainable standard for most people. He is also male, white and heterosexual, thus unrepresentative of a number of people with disability who experience double discrimination.

However, it is possible that the depiction of disability on a television show gave people an '"alibi" for discussion of … loaded topics' such as disability (Gray, 2008, p. 114). While Gray argues that depictions on fictional programs provide people an opportunity to consider shifting notions of reality, Turner (2009) identifies reality television as a format particularly suited to a mode of consumption whereby audiences feel more qualified to discuss the authenticity of a particular representation (p. 42).

Reality Television

Since the last major theorisation of disability on television, there have been significant developments regarding television, including the emergence of new genres such as reality television, home improvement programming, medical dramas, spin-off programming and websites that act as companions to television viewing. Coinciding with the surge in quality drama of which *Friday Night Lights* is indicative, reality TV emerged as a broadly popular television genre that could be made relatively cheaply (Sepinwall, 2012, p. 4). Aspects of these programs, which foreground the relevance of impairment and disability to the lives of people with disability, potentially advance social understandings of disability.

Reality television is a television-specific hybrid genre that draws on the conventions of a number of existing genres such as news and current affairs, documentary, docu-soap, soap opera, talk shows and game shows. It also draws on the intersection between voyeurism and cultural entertainment that has both preceded and encompassed the media, of which disability has played a major role. Reality TV continues the public's interest in visual stimulation which, historically, can be traced through the wealthy touring insane asylums and homes for the disabled during 1700s, to the popularity of wax museums of the 1800s, to freak shows popular between 1840 and 1940 where people with disabilities were displayed as human curiosities.

As these forms of popular culture have been replaced by the media, and particularly television, reality television programming has embraced characters with disability for a similar mode of visual stimulation and emotional appeal. Natalie Wilson (2005) argues that gay, black and disabled bodies are strategically placed on reality TV. These strategic placements often feature in talent contest reality TV formats such as *The Voice, Britain's Got Talent, The X Factor,* the *Idol* franchise (e.g. *Pop Idol, American Idol, Australian Idol* etc.), *Project Runway, America's Next Top Model* and *Masterchef.* The inclusion of such characters with disability in reality TV is frequently criticised as reinforcing a discourse of normality based on a 'white, able-bodied, heteronormative paradigm' (Wilson, 2005, p. 7).

Dave Calvert describes 2009 *Britain's Got Talent* contestant Susan Boyle as the first 'learning disabled celebrity' to attract international mainstream media attention (Calvert, 2013, p. 1). He argues that the media and audience reaction to Boyle reveals the ways impairments are constructed as disability in discourse. As I discuss further in Chapter 8, Boyle's audition is an important moment in popular culture as we transition from a broadcast environment to spreadable media (Jenkins, 2013). While the initial broadcast performance was edited for maximum emotional resonance, its spread across web platforms such as YouTube was the result of grassroots fan decisions. As Boyle was turned into spreadable content she received international attention.

Reality television competition style programs include participants with disability in order to boost ratings by eliciting an emotional response in the audience. Often these competitors engage in the requisite discourse, namely that, although they do not want to be seen as the disabled competitor, the judges then proceed to construct them as exactly that. For example, when Emmanuel Kelly, a refugee with vision impairment, competed in *Australia's Got Talent*, the judges focused only on his back story, rather than talent. However, as Graeme Turner argues, this is keeping with the broader tendency of this genre where contestants ostensibly audition for an opportunity for career progression yet, instead of focusing on their talent, they argue their case in terms of their 'essential selves' (Turner, 2009, p. 3). The role of disability in this 'recognition of the self' cannot be ignored.

Proceeding from Mitchell and Snyder's body genres introduced in the previous chapter, reality television as a television specific genre relies on disability to elicit emotion from the audience. A leaked casting memo from *Extreme Makeover: Home Edition* uncovered by the Smoking Gun revealed the producers' search for families affected by a number of specific impairments from Muscular Dystrophy to Down's Syndrome to ALS, propgeria, congenital insensitivity to pain with antidrodis (CIPA), and skin cancer (The Smoking Gun, 2006). For Jonathan Gray, this memo and the program itself where 'a sad story of an afflicted family' whose suffering is eased by 'completely rebuilding and redesigning their home' demonstrates the televisual process of 'normalization in action' (Gray, 2008, p. 160). With the defining message of reality television in general being 'overcoming the odds', narratives concerning people with disability hyperbolise the concept.

Despite this, reality TV also offers the opportunity for more diverse representations of disability (Wilde and Williams, 2011; Müller, Klijn et al., 2012). While early seasons of *Big Brother* demonstrated a lack of body diversity, later seasons have included several housemates with disabilities (Wilde and Williams, 2011). Müller, Klijn and Van Zoonen argue that reality television may therefore educate people with little experience with disability through both incidentalist and non-incidentalist strategies of representation. Contestants with disabilities such as *Masterchef*'s Christine Ha, whose use of assistive technologies was depicted throughout the series, and *Project Runway*'s Justin LeBlanc, who was provided accommodations including an interpreter, illustrate their argument that reality television may also offer a new template for media representations of disability by recognising the intersection between the impairment of the body and a disabling society.

Push Girls

The reality TV series *Push Girls* offers a further innovation of the character with disability in a reality TV show format. The series follows four glamorous and empowered LA women with disability from diverse ethnicities, sexualities and perspectives on living with disability – Tiphany, Angela, Auti and Mia.

A progression of disability representation can be discerned throughout season 1 of this series. While early episodes may embrace an overly sympathetic, wondrous and inspirational tone in order to capture an audience, later episodes introduce important disability critiques. Even more important than this representation, however, is the way both fans and antifans (people who do not watch the show, including those who flatly refuse to) use the show to discuss disability as socially and culturally situated. Like *Friday Night Lights*, the narrative introduces issues associated with community and sexuality – topics also taken up in the online discussion.

Executive producer Gay Rosenthal, who also produces *Little People Big World* had originally wanted to create a reality series about Angela Rockwood, who prior to becoming quadriplegic had a role in *The Fast and the Furious*, focusing on her relationship with husband Dustin Nguyen, of *21 Jump Street* fame, but upon meeting Angela's friends Tiphany, Mia and Auti shifted focus to 'the girls' . She describes *Push Girls* as a show about 'four girlfriends juggling dating and babies and careers. Their lives are interesting, with a dramatic twist' (Rosenthal cited in Kusler, 2012). The series begins with Tiphany, a conventionally attractive blonde, explaining the way people stare at people with disability:

> Los Angeles is definitely a body conscious place to live. After I first got injured
> I used to be so shy and insecure because everyone stared. Some people would
> just come straight out and ask "what's wrong with you?" …

She juxtaposes this feeling of dis-ease with the assertion that now she loves attention and has never been in better shape. Her voice over accompanies vision of her flirting with an attractive man while filling her car with petrol. In this scene Tiphany connotes the to-be-looked-at-ness I discussed in Chapter 3 and

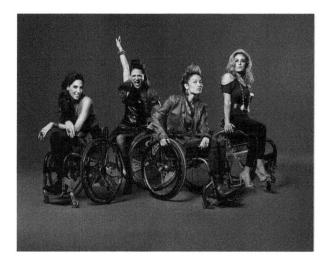

Figure 5.2 ***Push Girls*: Mia Schaikewitz, Auti Angel, Angela Rockwood, Tiphany Adams**

Source: © JC Dhien courtesy of SundanceTV.

the good -looking stranger gazes at her as opposed to stares at her disability. She, however, controls the gaze and turns him into an object for her visual pleasure:

> It's been almost 10 years now that I've been in a wheelchair … I do not have a hard time getting attention, I love flirting …. I have 26 inch rims on the side of my arse. It's hard not to get attention. (S1 E1)

The episode continues by chronicling the traumatic onsets of the women's impairments against an emotionally searing soundtrack. Tiphany explains she was involved in a drunk-driving accident and was pronounced dead at the scene; in a later episode she reveals she was only given a 5 per cent chance of surviving to the next week. Angela, also the series producer, recounts her own traumatic car accident and is the only quadriplegic in the group. Archival footage of Auti as a back-up dancer to hip hop artist LL Cool J is juxtaposed with images of her wheelchair dancing in her living room. She also explains that she was involved in a car accident, with the added trauma of it occurring immediately after she prostituted herself to pay her bills, despite having just danced back-up at the Grammys. The last of the 'four', Mia, explains that she was a swimming champion who became paralysed over the course of a day after suffering a ruptured blood vessel in her spinal cord at the age of 15. While these descriptions are repeated almost verbatim throughout the first few episodes of the series and follow the personal tragedy discourse of disability, adjusting to life as a person with disability is an important theme that runs throughout the series. While the four main cast members are depicted as secure in their identities as women, the notion that this has not always been the case is explored through newer cast member Chelsea who at 19 is much younger than the women and has only recently experienced her injury, also in a drunk-driving accident, two years prior.

A robust and energetic online discussion between both fans and antifans has emerged around *Push Girls*. While promotional material and statements made in the program itself attempt to reposition disability within discourses of beauty and femininity, the show has received considerable social media criticism for perpetuating an either/or image of disability (see H. McKay, 2013). The social media criticism emerged in direct response to a comment Tiphany made in the first episode, that she wanted to dispel the stereotype that women in wheelchairs were dirty and stayed at home wearing sweats while playing video games. In the case of *Push Girls*, regardless of whether people watched the program or not, the activity of social networking had the larger aim of creating a more accessible and diverse community that would include people with disability.

Online audiences discussing the show variously identify as fans, antifans, disabled, non-disabled and, at times, unable to afford the cable subscription or the additional cost of captioning services on catch-up television. Their discussion reveals several insights regarding the position of people with disability in society. Firstly, regardless of whether people identified as fans or antifans, all expressed an interest in increasing the representation of people with disability in the media and in television entertainment in particular. There was disagreement, however, regarding how to do this – while some focused on the 'they just happen to be in wheelchairs' angle, others pointed out that, at times, having a disability is hard, particularly when locations are inaccessible and attitudes disabling.

In addition to issues related to social disablement, *Push Girls* offers insight into what Carol Thomas (1999) describes as impairment effects. While the plot lines ascribe closely to the types of narratives common in women's genre such as relationships, career and the decision to start a family, the effects of the women's impairments impacts on almost every part of their lives, revealing that having a disability requires more than a 'good attitude'. For example, when discussing blind dates and abusive relationships, Auti, Tiphany and Mia comment on the increased vulnerability of being in a wheelchair. When Auti investigates the possibility of having children, her doctor goes through risk factors such as blood clots that women with paralysis must take into account.

Participants in the popular Television Without Pity (TWOP) discussion forums recognise the 'universal challenges' faced by these women:

Conceiving a child. Finding new employment. Being separated from a spouse. Trying to have a mature relationship with a parent. Deciding whether a relationship is supportive or stifling. By focusing on those problems, and not really so much the wheel-chair issues, the show really becomes one about women facing problems we all have and can relate to. (ThatGrrl comment on maraleia, 2012)

The stares of others is a theme that appears throughout this series and the tag line 'if you can't stand up, stand out' suggests these women invite – and indeed control – the stare. Later in the series Angela recounts her acronym ('PS') for the attention this group of wheelchair users receive whenever they are out together – 'people staring'. However, through participation in a reality TV series they reclaim this stare, giving people permission to look but only under certain restrictions.

In episode 9 'Freaky Deaky', the four women go out to an art gallery where they attract an inordinate amount of attention. This attention oscillates between the type of attention attractive women receive in public spaces and awe and wonder that people with disability leave the house. Seeing one person with disability at an art gallery may attract the stares of others, but four beautiful and glamorous women together seems quite unusual. While Mia comments on the ways people are looking at them rather than the art in the gallery, she and Tiphany are accused of faking their disabilities. *Push Girls* leverages this stare as an opportunity to comment on life with a disability, revealing the way the attitudes of others adversely affects people with disability. Mia in particular is enraged by the accusation that she is not disabled, speaking to camera – 'I wanted to run after him and grab him and find out what he was thinking and why he said that. Obviously ignorance'.

However, the series has a strong affiliation with the Reeve–Irvine Research Center, whose focus on cure has been criticised by disability activists, academics and commentators. In episode 6, 'Fired Up', Angela decides to visit the centre and talk to Dr Oswald about current discoveries in spinal research. He tells Angela that he believes there will be a cure in her lifetime. This particular claim was debated by both fans and antifans following a review of the episode posted by Tiffany Carlson on *Beauty Ability*. The participants on *Beauty Ability* explore a number of relevant themes and issues such as coming to terms with acquired disability, making choices after injury, and the idea that there is not one universal experience of disability. It also considers the limitations of *Push Girls* as a forum for presenting such issues, further evidence of the same discussion appearing in popular culture, and the ethics of the topic of stem cell surgery and the (what some saw as empty) promises that surround it (see Carlson, 2012).

The episode itself offers a broader debate about stem cell research. The episode begins by once again positioning the girls as attractive and sexualised women through close ups on Mia's legs and face – in an example of what Laura Mulvey described as festishisation and then moves on to Mia and Tiphany at the gym, where they discuss working out to the point of exhaustion and make statements to the camera about the importance of physical fitness. The episode then focuses on a disagreement among the group regarding stem cell research. While Chelsea – who is shown participating in a form of physiotherapy called Project Walk – is enthusiastic about potentially participating in stem cell surgery to regain the ability to walk, Mia and Auti are against it. Whereas Auti cites ethical reasons, Mia says she hates society's focus on 'fixing' people so that they are perfect. Angela, who has actually had stem cell surgery, comments to the camera that Mia and Auti's argument is 'BS'. The episode provides a number of perspectives on the issue which Auti describes as dividing the wheelchair community.

'Fired Up' also comments on the ways people with disability are presented as inspirational. With the older women trying to encourage Chelsie to see her disablement as having a higher inspirational purpose, she asks 'what does that do for me physically?' She professes a strong desire to walk and says she doesn't think it's fair that she was the only person in her car accident that didn't get a second chance to walk. In response to further encouragement that she's inspiring and helping people, Chelsie points out 'You've helped so many people, I've helped so many people but who has helped us?'

In *The Cinema of Isolation* Martin Norden comments on the ways women with disability have been constructed onscreen as not 'marriage material' (p. 21). *Push Girls* both acknowledges and rejects this stereotype. Chelsea voices the concerns of the general population that acquiring a disability signals the end of one's sex life when she comments that the boys she would have previously 'got' with a click of her fingers would not even look twice at her now. The women in *Push Girls* comment on the way this attitude affects their dating lives, with people encouraging them to 'settle'. Mia in particular rejects this notion. In season 1 she breaks up with her boyfriend of one and a half years because he does not want to have children and refuses second dates with two men with whom she doesn't feel a 'spark'. Both Tiphany and Mia have active dating lives and are shown speed dating, approaching men in bars and attracting the attention of men in the street. Similarly, Tiphany frequently discusses her sex life, specifically her ability to have 'lots and lots and lots of sex', and her propensity to attract attention from interested men. Participants in the TWOP forum criticise Tiphany's constant references to her sex life and instead describe Auti and her husband Eric's relationship as a positive representation of marriage on television and applaud their conversations and issues as being man/woman discussions not able/disabled.

Angela, who has separated from her husband, embarks on a new relationship in the second half of the first season. Whereas television usually hides the messiness of female bodily functions from view and in particular obscures this aspect of embodiment from any narrative involving dating, in *Push Girls*, Angela must teach her new boyfriend Cody to catheterise her in order to go away for a weekend together. The trip is significant because Angela is attending her first modelling job since becoming disabled and, in order to take Cody as her romantic partner and have some time alone together, he must also act as her carer.

Angela, Cody, Auti, Mia, Tiphany and Angela's carer Aunt Judy offer a sort of round table of relevant views and differing perspectives on Angela's decision to ask Cody to care for her on the trip. It is clearly not an easy decision for anyone. While Auti is concerned because 'all of your parts down there are supposed to be sexy. When your man is your caregiver, it kind of ruins that', Mia adds that 'there's a fine line between boyfriends and caregivers. In Angela's case though, it's sometimes inevitable that your significant other will have to be that'. Angela describes herself as 'a high maintenance 125 pound baby' who needs help going to the toilet. Judy expresses concern that Cody won't be able to offer adequate care, while Cody himself comments that he prefers to have a nurse around. Tiphany, however, is confident that Cody will 'man up'.

While *Push Girls* has been positively reviewed and received a critic's choice award, it has also received a significant amount of social media criticism, particularly for its focus on beauty and tragedy. The series has been criticised for perpetuating the beauty myth through its use of conventionally beautiful glamorous youthful disabled women who do not have to deal with messy aspects of impairment:

Triumph over tragedy, always makes for good TV. Every voyeur's fetish about people with impairments is facilitated. Minimised and modified – dainty wheelchairs with the delicacy of haute couture clothes – impairments – in a shiny, neat package. (McDonagh, 2013)

The scene in which Angela engages a photographer to begin rebuilding her modelling portfolio reinforces a 'triumph-over-tragedy' representation, however contradictions and questions are also introduced. Whereas Angela approaches the meeting with the intention of demonstrating that she is still able to model, albeit in a slightly different way, the photographer looks perplexed for most of the shoot, and especially when Angela's leg goes into spasm. He later describes her as like the baseball pitcher with no hands. Yet the comparison does not make sense because Angela has a beautiful face and is seeking out headshots for 'beauty' work.

Although *Push Girls* is an example of progressive television, the issues that McDonagh raises – particularly around the emergence of a new beauty myth that further marginalises people with 'messier' impairments – must be kept in mind. We should also question the eagerness of applying damaging discourses of beauty to all women, specifically to women with disability as an example of empowerment. Both Angela and Tiphany are models, while Auti, Mia and Chelsea are dancers. Leroy Moore criticises this feature of the show:

> I was glad to see that there are at least two woman of color and all of them are real women with disabilities, but for me it's not enough and it's not anything new. Of course, all of them fall into the mainstream media's stereotypical image of a woman that we always see on T.V.: skinny, white or light skin, etc. (Moore, 2012)

Moore – who is highly critical of the show to the point of not watching beyond the first couple of episodes – fits Gray's (2008) definition of the antifan. His criticism of *Push Girls'* lack of disability politics and awareness of disability history is an example of the political nature of antifandom in the way it reveals 'our individual and communal criteria for what television should be' (Gray, 2008, p. 62).

Conclusion

Television provides an insight into people, environments and situations that we otherwise might not have any experience with. Although the numbers of characters with a disability on television remain unacceptably low, and television representation does in some cases perpetuate prejudice against people with disabilities, people with disabilities now dominate a number of formats and genres. Examples include dramas (*Friday Night Lights, The West Wing, Glee, CSI, Parenthood, Hannibal, Beverly Hills 90210, Homeland*), comedies (*Becker, The Last Leg, Life's Too Short, Big Bang Theory,*), sport (*The Olympics, The Paralympics*), advertising (Apple, Doritos, Dove, Guinness), and reality television (*Britain's Missing Top Model, Push Girls, Take a Seat, Masterchef, Project Runway*). In addition to these main characters with disabilities, television dramas and comedies now regularly feature people with disabilities in minor roles.

However, following research that took place in 1988, Guy Cumberbatch and Ralph Negrine argued that people with disabilities were poorly underrepresented on television. They found that people with disabilities were mainly represented in 'factual' programming, crime dramas and film and posited that, in order for social change to occur, people with disabilities needed to become 'amongst the leading characters on television' (Cumberbatch and Negrine, 1992, p. 140). They needed to be shown as 'ordinary' people with ordinary problems. However, British disability theorist Colin Barnes was not as optimistic in his review of their book *Images of Disability on Television*, and criticised Cumberbatch and Negrine for failing to interrogate the ways 'television is instrumental in perpetuating disabled people's oppression'. However, Barnes' distinctly social model approach does not take into consideration the workings of television as popular culture, as a producerly text. It can be argued that, where television fails as a radical text, it succeeds as a progressive one. As Fiske suggests, we should turn to analysis of popular texts to 'expose their contradictions, their meanings that escape control, their producerly intentions' (Fiske, 1989, 2010, p. 85). Similarly, Fiske recognises that, despite reinforcing the status quo, some meanings escape control and that television reflects a progression of social values.

Following Fiske's framework of the producerly text, this chapter undertook an assessment of disability on television to consider moments of resistance in the way disability figures on television as popular culture. Although disability theorists have most often focused on the incorporation of disability under the dominant framework, certain elements escape hegemonic control and reveal that a struggle does exist for greater social inclusion.

Chapter 6
Enfreaking Popular Music: Making Us Think by Making Us Feel

Def Leppard drummer Rick Allen severed his arm when he crashed his Corvette driving to a New Year's Eve party in 1984. Allen's arm was eventually amputated following an infection. In order to continue playing drums for the hard rock band – who went on to significant popular success with songs such as *Hysteria* and *Love Bites* – Allen collaborated with engineers and other musicians to create an electronic drum kit that allowed his left foot to operate the snare, enabling him to play drums one handed. He also established the Raven Drum Foundation and the One Hand Drum Company to support people going through crisis.

Music journalist Mick Middles described Joy Division's Ian Curtis as a 'twitching epileptic-like mass of flesh and bone' in his 1979 review of one of the seminal Manchester band's gigs (cited in G. McKay, 2013, p. 113). Curtis did in fact have epilepsy, and, despite having seizures onstage and making reference to epilepsy in 'She's Out of Control', fans were reportedly unaware of the condition until several years after his death (Waltz and James, 2009). His wife Deborah Curtis described his onstage dancing as a 'distressing parody of his offstage seizures' (cited in G. McKay, 2013, p. 113). However, his epilepsy has since become a key marketing feature of the band's enduring influence, and Curtis, who previously worked with people with disability and eventually committed suicide, is a central figure of the cultural discourse of the tortured artist.

In 2013 *The Guardian* reported that Lady Gaga had commissioned New York designer Ken Borochov to create a 'bejewelled wheelchair' for her personal use as she recovered from hip surgery (Michaels, 2013). The pop artist has consistently drawn on themes and images related to disability, enfreakment and social marginalisation such as wheelchairs and canes in her music videos, stage performances, pop persona and promotional images – and has been heavily criticised in the disability blogosphere for it. Although she does not identify as disabled, she invokes the discourse of the freak show and monstrous other as part of her identity and has spoken publically of her experiences with impairment, claiming to have been diagnosed 'borderline lupus' in 2010 (Miserandino, 2010) and later undergoing hip surgery.

Although it has gone unrecognised, disability and music have long been intertwined. Colin Cameron's (2009) definition of disability culture as 'a site within which social and positional identities are struggled for and dominant discourses rejected' (p. 381) is evident throughout the history of disability in popular music. Whereas Cameron refers explicitly to disability-specific counter-cultural music forms, similar tendencies can be seen throughout the history of disability's influence on pop. For example, Anthony Tusler (2005) notes the impact disability and impairment have had on the composition of a number of popular songs – from a disabled veteran begging his partner to remain faithful in the 1960s' pop song *Ruby Don't Take Your Love to Town,* to Joey Ramone's OCD influencing the Ramones' *Cretin Hop.* However, it is George McKay's recent monograph *Shakin' All Over: Popular Music and Disability* that provides the first comprehensive examination of disability in popular music from a post-social and cultural model of disability. McKay (2013) argues that disability is foundational to popular music and makes the observation that disability and the popular music industry emerged *at the same time* (p. 3). McKay links the social construction of disability with the emergence of the concept of normal during the nineteenth and twentieth centuries and historicises disability's influence on popular music in relation to modernity, the mass media and popular culture. This chapter takes up his project through a critical analysis of Lady Gaga as a contemporary example of the mutual importance of disability to popular music and popular music to disability.

Popular culture – and popular music especially – is often accused of being formulaic, of pandering to a mass audience, and of occupying a lower status to so-called high culture. With the history of popular music characterised by moments of resistance and incorporation, the image of disability and the ways it is used to elicit emotion illustrate a shifting cultural mindset.

Although a burgeoning music focused sub-field of critical disability studies has emerged and is gaining traction, *popular* music is undertheorised. This chapter applies observations from music disability studies (see Lubet, 2011) and cultural investigations of the freak show to explore the significance of disability using the example of Lady Gaga's popular music and freak aesthetic in prompting her audiences to both think and feel about the non-normative. Although analysis of musical lyrics and composition is important, in analysing a pop music personality such as Lady Gaga, the discussion must extend to a consideration of the pop persona, especially in the current converging and digitised media environment where celebrities appear in music videos and communicate directly with their fans on social networking sites such as Facebook and Twitter. I further expand this discussion to consider the specific ways in which Lady Gaga's fans and antifans creatively produce their own related content and cultural critique.

Pop superstar Lady Gaga represents an important moment in popular music. Her name is an ironic reference to Queen's 1984 song *Radio Ga Ga*, yet her persona leverages new participatory and digital cultures. Tara Brabazon and Steve Redhead (2013) argue that her significance as a text within popular cultural studies goes beyond case study, for Lady Gaga is a 'metaphor, metonymy, and model' to think about pop's past, present and future which, as a result of digitisation, is accelerating exponentially – Lady Gaga achieved in under 5 years what took other pop artists decades.

Disability and Music

In the introduction to their edited collection *Sounding Off: Theorizing Disability in Music*, Joseph Straus and Neil Lerner (2006) argue that music, like history and literature, has a number of stories to tell about disability. In her foreword to the collection, Garland-Thomson (2006) observes that disability appears in music under four broad categories. The first concerns 'disability themes' in music. From themes about stuttering, popular between 1890 and the 1930s (see Goldmark, 2006), to a number of more recent critiques of psychiatric institutions (see Abby jean, 2010a, 2010b), disability is a topic that features in music. Secondly, Garland-Thomson recognises that disability may impact on musical performance. A number of theorists have noted the disabling significance of impairment on musicians who rely on their bodies to create their art (Cain, 2010; Lubet, 2011), while others note the influence of impairment on the artist's work itself (Church, 2006; Headlam, 2006; Morrison and Finkelstein, 1997). These impacts can be seen in both the works of Allen and Curtis introduced at the beginning of the chapter. While Allen made use of adaptive technologies to continue performing as a drummer, Curtis became known for his distinctive dancing, which in some cases could have been seizures.

The third area of study that Garland-Thomson identifies is an interrogation of the signification of disability in music. Although the question of what the performer is trying to communicate in their signification of disability is particularly important in the post music video era where songs with and without disability themes now feature disability imagery, the incorporation of people with disabilities as props in live performances – such as Miley Cyrus' dwarf backup dancers – begs a similar question.

Finally, Garland-Thomson suggests we consider the ways disability structures music. Garland-Thomson comments that we are trained to think of disability as a medical condition and that this acculturation informs musical production. She recommends an exploration of the ways disability shapes music and, by extension, the ways music shapes disability. Elspeth Morrison and Vic Finklestein (1997) agree and comment that, when disabled musicians are recognised, their lives are usually 'seen in terms of their medical condition and their imagined ability to overcome personal tragedy' (p. 161). Celia Cain (2010) attributes this to the cliché that 'great art requires great sacrifice'. Outlining common examples of this, from Beethoven's deafness to Kurt Cobain's suicide, she comments that music scholarship has avoided disability except through 'romanticized tropes of tragic artists' (p. 747).

She further identifies a pressure on musicians to 'pass' as non-disabled and pain-free in order to alleviate the cultural 'fear of contagion' (Cain, 2010, p. 750). She maintains that a fear of disablement pervades musicians who make use of their body for art. As a result, the cultural story of heroes overcoming adversary is retold as a way to seek comfort in a community of 'sacrificing' artists. Some commentators have accused Lady Gaga of fabricating her hip injury to leverage this cultural script (see Celeb Daily News, 2013). Indeed, her participation in and subversion of the culture of passing was revealed when she cancelled the remaining 20 shows of her tour the Born This Way Ball via Facebook and Twitter in February 2013, and is evidence of pop's ongoing fascination with passing and sacrificing artists:

> There's an unfortunate announcement coming out right now, concerning myself and the Born This Way Ball. Im so sorry. I barely know what to say. I've been hiding a show injury and chronic pain for sometime now, over the past month it has worsened. I've been praying it would heal. I hid it from my staff, I didn't want to disappoint my amazing fans. However after last nights performance I could not walk and still can't. (Lady Gaga, 2013)

Yet disability and popular music continues to be undertheorised. A 2009 special issue of the journal *Popular Music* remains one of the only comprehensive investigations of this area. Papers in the issue consider diverse topics such as disability as a marketing strategy, with reference to Joy Division (Waltz and James, 2009), the emergence of a disability arts counter music culture in Britain in the 1980s (C. Cameron, 2009), and the cultural mediation of Johnny Ray (Herr, 2009). George McKay, who edited this special issue, continues his argument in *Shakin' All Over* that disability is everywhere in popular music and reveals a history of disability in popular music.

While McKay describes his approach to disability in popular music as a cripping of music and a popping of disability, his observations around the presence of disability in popular music is similar to Garland-Thomson's argument that disability appears in music under the four categories of themes, impact on performance, signification and structure. McKay's focus on the pop persona as it is constructed and managed within the popular music industry adds a fifth dimension to the analysis. His discussion of The Who exploring and returning to tropes of disability over its long career is particularly illustrative:

The Who stuttered the attitudinal voice of English youth in 1964's "My Generation" ("People try to put us d-d-down"), sang and acted "That deaf dumb and blind kid [who] sure plays a mean pinball" in the film *Tommy* in 1975, while guitarist Pete Townshend was widely reported when he spoke out recently about the experience and dangers of rock-music-induced hearing loss. (G. McKay, 2013, p. 11)

This brief history of the significance of disability across The Who's career from 'youthful stutter to hearing impairment' demonstrates the dominating structure of disability in terms of themes, impact on performance and signification. The general fascination with otherness evident in The Who's body of work and pop persona is also reflected in the popular music industry more generally.

McKay locates the origins of a disability presence in popular music within the polio epidemic in much of the Western world and situates Ian Dury at the centre of 'a strand of disabled cultural identity' (p. 46). Dury – the lead singer of the iconic 1970s/'80s English group the Blockheads – suffered polio as a child and sang of his experiences with institutionalisation and social disablement. McKay argues that Dury forms the bridge between earlier popular artists with disability such as Gene Vincent and the figure of post-punk enfreakment in the hunchbacked body of Johnny Rotten of the Sex Pistols.

Like Vincent, Dury and Rotten, Lady Gaga celebrates the freakish in her creation of a new pop aesthetic. Like The Who she has explored and returned to tropes of disability throughout her career, from encouraging her father to have heart surgery in 'Speechless' ('could we fix you if you broke?'), to invoking the image of disability in her *Paparazzi* video to critique celebrity culture, to extending the critique of 'the brutalized feminine' (Brabazon and Redhead, 2013) in a disabling homage to Madonna's *Like a Virgin* video in her 2009 VMA performance. Disability has also appeared onstage as a wheelchair-using mermaid, in promotional videos where Lady Gaga becomes cyborg like, and through her own impairment and recuperation, necessitating time away from the industry.

The Emotional Intensification of the Freak Show: An Opportunity for Transgressive Reappropriation?

Provoking an emotional reaction from spectators and audiences is a defining characteristic of number of forms of popular culture, from Soviet film director and theorist Sergei Eisenstein's 1920s' theory of attractions, to arcade game designers seeking to capture gamer interest in under 2 minutes, to freak show performances and music videos. Henry Jenkins (2007) describes this as the 'wow climax', and observes that it is one of the most denigrated features of popular culture. The distinction between high and popular culture often views the popular as a cultural wasteland that can only ever confirm 'cultural decline or the need for regulation and social control' (Storey, 2003, p. 31). Jenkins further locates this distinction in the realm of emotion:

> Most popular culture is shaped by a logic of emotional intensification. It is less interested in making us think than it is in making us feel. Yet that distinction is too simple: popular culture, at its best, makes us think by making us feel. (Jenkins, 2007, p. 3)

He argues that while popular culture can get by using 'well-trod formulas', the most successful popular culture elicits a 'wow climax' from its audience. This response relies on broadly shared cultural feelings that reveal central cultural 'conflicts, anxieties, fantasies, and fears' (Jenkins, 2007, p. 3). While Jenkins does not refer to the freak show, he highlights the enduring significance of the circus showman and sideshow performer to popular culture's quest for an emotional reaction. These performers had to attract and maintain a mass audience; for Jenkins, the spectacle was based on aesthetic, not storytelling.

The freak show and vaudeville circus is a culturally significant form of entertainment which raises several uncomfortable questions around enfreakment and the employment and exploitation of people with disability. However, as Robert Bogdan argued in *Freak Show: Presenting Human Oddities for Amusement and Profit*, '"Freak" is a frame of mind, a set of practices, a way of thinking about and presenting people' (p. 3). While freak shows may have exhibited 'human oddities', they were stylised to appear that way, for example giants or the obese would appear with very small furniture to look larger than they really were. Similarly, General Tom Thumb, one of the more famous dwarf freak show performers claimed to be five years old when he was actually 11. Deception and misrepresentation leveraged the perceived deviance of the performers – rather than attempt any assistance to move society past that discomfort towards greater social inclusion – and was central to the freak show performance. The freak show thus becomes a clear site of cultural construction.

While freak shows are now considered bad taste and have been criticised by disability theorists, cultural historians and medical practitioners, some disability theorists have identified transgressive features of the format. Although David Gerber (1996) argues that freak show scholarship should only condemn freak shows (p. 43), a number of works introduce important investigations of the freak show, enfreakment and freak performance (Barnes, 1997; Bogdan, 1990; Garland-Thomson, 1996; Gerber, 1996; Hevey, 1992). For example, Bogdan, with whom Gerber takes direct issue, argues that in addition to degradation and demeaning representations, people with disability also featured in freak shows in 'ways that positively enhanced their status' (Bogdan, 1990, p. viii). Further, Michael Chemer's (2005) observations that freak scholarship is emerging as a 'lineage of serious writings which investigate freakery not solely as the victimisation of a disenfranchised minority but rather as a highly specialised and potentially liberatory form of performance art' holds significance for both writerly and producerly performances of disability. The freak show has become an important site for transgressive reappropriation or the reusing of problematic images in a more progressive way. This has also been reflected in popular culture and music, especially with performers such as Lady Gaga and Michael Jackson – particularly his character representation in the *Thriller* video as well as his at times bizarre offstage behaviour– embracing a reappropriation of the freak.

Words such as freak and monster pervade Lady Gaga's transmedia pop persona. Whereas her fans call themselves 'little monsters' and Gaga herself 'mother monster', in an act of transgressive reappropriation Lady Gaga invites people to engage with her music as fellow freaks, outsiders, outcasts and people who are otherwise misunderstood. She describes her embrace of difference and how she seeks to encourage her fans to accept themselves for who they are:

> The best thing about The Monster Ball is that I created it so that my fans have a place to go. A place where all the freaks are outside and I lock the fucking doors. It doesn't matter who you are … because tonight and every night after you could be whoever it is that you want to be. (Gagapedia, 2010)

In interviews she explains that she wants her community of fans to feel as though they have a 'freak in me to hang out with and they don't feel alone' (Lady Gaga cited in Corona, 2011, p. 726). She invokes the discourse of the freak show to problematise the cultural focus on perfection. She expresses desire to offer a space of inclusion for her fans whom she sees as socially excluded by mainstream culture:

> My fanbase are people from different backgrounds, different sexual orientations, different music tastes, they're all dressed up like they're going to see *Rocky Horror Picture Show* … It's a creative decision with my fashion to be androgynous and scary. (Lady Gaga cited in Arjan, 2008)

Her œuvre also recognises the history of popular culture and draws inspiration from other acts which celebrate difference or offer performances of abnormality as entertainment. Lady Gaga's focus on transgression, identity politics and otherness position her as a key figure in popular social change discourse. She also constantly uses the tools of pop culture to reinvent her appearance, and builds upon and breaks existing formulas to offer a critique of cultural ideals of pop music discourses of feminine perfection. Lady Gaga's pursuit of the feminine ideal is not natural, nor ideal (see Gray, 2012). Celebrity freaks push boundaries of normality and behave in ways that do not always make sense. For David Yuan (1996), celebrities such as Michael Jackson who appropriate the freakish as a site of 'theatricalized transgression' draw attention to the cultural value that is arbitrarily applied to physical features of the body (p. 368).

Lady Gaga: Performing Difference, Critiquing Perfection

Born Stefani Germanotta, Lady Gaga released her first single *Just Dance* in 2008. *Rolling Stone* described her as the 'the biggest new pop star of 2009' in the first half of that year (Hiatt, 2009). By 2010 she was the most Googled celebrity in the US (Corona, 2011) and had been named in the top 10 of the world's most powerful women (A. Cameron, 2012). At the time of writing she has over one billion social media followers on Facebook and Twitter.

For Brabazon and Redhead (2013), Lady Gaga is a layered text who 'loops, folds, changes, and transforms' diverse acts and performers from Queen, Elton John, Donna Summers, Madonna, Debbie Harry and David Bowie in a 'self-made bricolage'. However, Lady Gaga, who has been heavily criticised as derivative of artists such as Madonna to the point of theft (see Paglia, 2010), is reflexive about her attempts to build on and break existing formulas:

> I reference constantly but I most recently felt that I have had some truly original moments and if you get one really good original moment in your career you're solid. (Lady Gaga cited in A. Cameron, 2012, p. 211)

Lady Gaga uses disability imagery to critique the dominant culture which excludes disability from discourses of beauty. She distinguishes herself from her pop contemporaries such as Beyoncé, Shakira and Britney Spears through a visual aesthetic that rejects appearing 'as perfect as possible' (Dilling-Hansen, 2012). Gaga explains:

> I don't feel that I look like the other perfect little pop singers. I think I look new. I think I'm changing what people think is sexy. (Lady Gaga cited in Hiatt, 2009)

Lady Gaga's success within popular culture rests on both her creation of a subcultural community and her appeal to mainstream audiences. Her music and style of dress question what is at the core of humanness. However, her series of promotional photographs with the photographer David LaChapelle elicited major criticisms from the disability community, as did her video for

Paparazzi and her performance at the 2009 MTV Video Music Awards. These three representations are connected as performances which embrace Chemers' (2005) definition of freakery, 'constructed abnormality as entertainment'. So, while it can be seen that Lady Gaga has been able to leverage a community of little monsters through her enfreakment and discourse of the social reject, critiques of her use of disability imagery are also readily available. Taken together, these images and arguments offer important, albeit contradictory, cultural perspectives on disability.

Disability Debates in/and Lady Gaga's Music Videos and Promotional Images

Music videos are the first original art form specific to broadcast television (Fiske, 1986). The format often lacks the cause and effect characteristic of narrative and instead celebrates style and excess. They can be difficult to follow in a narrative sense. In the post music video era where music that is not necessarily disability-themed *becomes* disability-themed through the use of disability imagery, the music video has become an important site of cultural mediation. For example vision impairment becomes a signifier for true love in Lionel Ritchie's 1984 video for *Hello*. Ritchie falls for a blind arts student who despite having never *seen* him, sculpts an exact likeness of his head. The music video is a particular cultural form that emphasises effect over cause, and signifier over signified in a celebration of excess and montage. In other words, the music video seeks out the wow climax.

Bad Romance *and David LaChapelle*

Richard Gray (2012) notes that 'Gaga's exhibitionism fundamentally flies in the face of normative trends by celebrating difference and deviance rather than likeness and conformity' (p. 55) and acknowledges the debt of Michael Jackson's *Thriller* monsters in Gaga's *Bad Romance* video. This video features Lady Gaga as a deformed sex slave who is sold to the Russian mafia. Similarly, her 2009 series of promotional photographs with David LaChapelle feature her melding with machines and nature. These images destabilise the 'perfect' human body. She appears cyborg like in all of the photos; one connects Gaga and a chrome wheelchair with beautiful pink flowers, another invokes scenes from *Metropolis* as she appears on a constructed city scape wearing metallic clothing, propped up by canes and surrounded by the dead naked bodies of men, women and babies with a blimp flying overhead and a spotlight shining down on them. The final image sees her hooked up to a machine and emitting electrical energy. Her large and matted hair is not unlike images of women performing in freak shows in the 1800s who 'soaked their hair in beer and teased it to make it frizz and stand up' (Frost, 1996, p. 257). These promotional photographs and the imagery in *Bad Romance* illustrate Dilling-Hansen's (2012) contention that 'Gaga destabilizes the category of human nature by suggesting humans might be closer to animals or machines than we like to think', a theme also explored in the science fiction films discussed in Chapter 4 and in disability performance art. These themes and imagery appear often in Lady Gaga's musical performances.

Paparazzi

Lady Gaga's video clip for *Paparazzi* is a critique of celebrity behaviour and betrayal and tabloid culture. The video follows a young starlet struggling with her rise to fame as she is hounded by the paparazzi and sold out by the people with whom she is most intimate. The video begins with Lady Gaga in bed with her lover; she asks him if he loves her, which he agrees that he does. Her insecurities are out of place among all the signifiers of fame and success within the room, including $100 bills with her face on them. The mood of the video shifts from a classic Hollywood romance film to a sort of porn/ snuff/paparazzi hybrid as her lover takes her outside, placing her in a precarious position on the edge of the balcony. Lady Gaga resists as her lover plays up to the camera, kissing her but looking at them. After a struggle captured in individual photos frames edited together as a montage, Lady Gaga falls from the heights of the balcony.

She is next seen exiting a limousine wearing a bejewelled neck brace. She is briefly pushed along in a wheelchair before standing with the aid of crutches. However, she remains 'disabled' only in the view of the paparazzi who cease paying attention to her. Throughout the rest of the video she is seen dancing and enacting revenge on the people who betrayed her – her maid and her lover. The paparazzi are only interested in Gaga to take photos of the dead bodies of the maid and lover, and later when she admits to killing her boyfriend. Thus the video is used to critique the paparazzi regarding their interest with behind-the-scenes drama rather than musical ability. This use of disability imagery could be read as a comment on the construction of the pop star. Consider for example the intense interest around Britney Spears' mental health and mothering abilities as opposed to her musical abilities in the period immediately preceding Gaga's ascent to fame.

The video is almost 8 minutes long and the so-called 'disability imagery' lasts for only 50 seconds. This imagery was discussed extensively in the disability blogosphere (Hamilton, 2009; Wade, 2010). Reactions to these images centred around three interrelated themes, including the idea that Gaga is both exploiting and glamorising the disabled and that the image of disability is utilised as part of a wider critique of Hollywood, the music industry and gossip journalism as being endemic with pathology. At the time, in among the disapproving blogs, comments and commentaries, there were some that suggested perhaps Lady Gaga had some kind of invisible disability, such as this comment from TheWhatIfGirl:

> I'm surprised that only one person in this entire thread seems to have even considered the idea that Lady Gaga herself might be disabled in some way. Not everyone's disabilities are visually evident, and those of us who aren't immediately evident tend to get a lot of crap for it when people do find out because we have supposedly been deceiving people since they didn't know we were FREAKS right away. (Wade, 2010)

While Anna Hamilton's original post in the online feminist magazine *Bitch!* conceded that a representation of disability in a music video was by itself 'somewhat promising' because disability is notoriously underrepresented in popular culture, in the conversational thread that followed, the author took an increasingly negative stance towards the imagery:

> LG's disability representation is troubling, even if it's not the entire point of the video. The fact that disability is used as a plot point and a prop is something that I think viewers should question, overall "point" of the video or no. I also do not appreciate her appropriation of disability to show the "messed up" ways in which celebrities are treated – to me, it smacks of appropriation without doing any actual questioning of how *actual people with disabilities* are treated. It strikes me as very surface-level. (Hamilton, 2009)

Others saw the use of disability in that video as an incorporation of disability into discourses of beauty, sexiness, glamour and the popular. As El Benito argues in another post:

> Lady Gaga's portrayal of people with "disability", whether temporary or not, is definitely "sexy". i don't care what anybody else says, LG is sexy and so is her video, as well as her position of being disabled. Firstly, that she can make a "disabled" person "sexy" is a good thing. Secondly, the whole costume accentuates the canes by making her look like "a mechanized robot". That would support the argument that the canes are simply for effect, yet that is not their only function. she uses her medium to greeat [sic] effect, in fact, and becomes one in essence with the canes. (Wade, 2010)

Lady Gaga's use of disability imagery was read as a critique of the dominant culture which excludes disability from discourses of beauty. To return to El Benito:

… her use of the wheelchair and the canes in her art at all is good thing for the disabled community, for it shows that major pop-stars, again, can be "sexy" though "disabled" and that is a positive message. (Wade, 2010)

A key feature of Lady Gaga's performances and persona is to distinguish herself from others by acknowledging that everything is a creation, that nothing about her image is natural. As I have discussed throughout this book, progressive counter-narratives of disability in popular culture can be seen in images which embrace sexualised imagery.

The final theme that emerged in the online criticism of Lady Gaga's 2009 use of disability imagery was that it was not a representation of disability, but rather a critique of the price of fame. This was a contentious argument, as disability bloggers sought to maintain a literal interpretation and instead focus on the damaging impacts of 'crip drag'. As previously mentioned, Lady Gaga invokes the images of the transgressive freak to push the boundaries of normality and to create a fan base of others who feel similarly socially isolated. These images are particularly transgressive for a young female pop artist promoting her music. Indeed, some commenters online read her use of disability imagery as a comment on the construction of the pop star. As jennyknopinski commented following Lisa Wade's article on *Sociologial Images*:

I always thought the disability imagery in Paparazzi was about how the public relishes seeing young, beautiful, famous women when they are impaired in some way. For example, the tabloid feeding-frenzies surrounding Britney Spears and her mental health issues or Lindsay Lohan and her addiction issues or Mary-Kate Olson and her eating disorder issues. We love a young hot woman, but we love her even more when there's something "wrong" with her. (Wade, 2010)

Marry the Night

The 2011 video of *Marry the Night* could be read as a response to these criticisms, as Lady Gaga reflects on her state of mind and the choices she makes regarding the placement of objects in videos. This could be interpreted as being about her life, psychological state and fame, a foray she admits within the video is entirely constructed:

When I look back on my life, it's not that I don't want to see things exactly as they happened, it's just that I prefer to remember them in an artistic way. And truthfully, the lie of it all is much more honest because I invented it.

She comments on the constructed nature of the video clip:

For example, those nurses they're wearing next season Calvin Klein, and so am I. And the shoes custom Giuseppe Zanotti. I tipped their gauze caps to the side like Parisian berets because I think it's romantic, and I also believe that mint will be very big in fashion next Spring.

The video is an exploration of Lady Gaga's desire to succeed and references scenes from *Fame* and *Flashdance* as shorthand for her own dance training in New York. The video comments on in/sanity and the hard work required to succeed while dealing with rejection and criticism. Lady Gaga describes her past as an 'unfinished painting' that she must make beautiful and tells a nurse who recalls delivering her as a newborn that she is going to be a star because she has nothing left to lose. The cause and effect is in a perpetual loop in this video.

Applause

In her recently released single *Applause*, Lady Gaga references popular culture from *Metropolis*, to Andy Warhol, to Madonna, to the silent German expressionist horror film *Dr Caligari*, to herself. At several points throughout the video Gaga appears as a jester in clown makeup. She claims that this is a reflection of the emotion she felt having been away from her fans for so long during her recuperation:

> I thought about nothing but my fans every minute since that tour ended. It was intense, especially because I'm such an active person and I love performing so much. It was challenging to stop performing. That was the hardest part, not seeing the fans, not performing, not playing the music. I'm not just a musician. I'm also a creative mind. It made it much more intense and amazing. Because I couldn't do anything else but create. I couldn't dance, I couldn't walk, so I created. I wrote all my ideas down every day. I obsessed over it. (Lady Gaga cited in ABC news, 2013)

Being unable to perform, or indeed walk, she describes rehearsing in her mind while lying down. Her experience recovering from hip surgery not only impacted on the composition of the song itself but also her music video performance. She describes the impact on her makeup and performance:

> We put this clown makeup on my face and as an ode to the jester. As I was performing on the set, I started to feel really emotional and sad because I hadn't seen my fans for a long time. It's very different performing for a camera than performing for 50,000 people. It feels different, and I truly miss them. So I took my hands and I smudged the makeup down my face like tears, and I began to cry while I was singing, singing, "I live for the applause". What I mean is not

that I live for attention, but I live for making them happy. And that's when the applause happens. When the audience loves it. (Lady Gaga cited in ABC news, 2013)

This observation recognises the importance of popular culture in eliciting an emotional response from the audience. The lyrics 'pop culture was in art; now art's in pop culture, in me' critique the distinction between high and popular culture as arbitrary and irrelevant. The video itself takes a number of signifiers of both high and popular culture and combines them in a display of pop culture excess. Taking Jenkins et al.'s (2002) argument that popular culture can be understood as a subversion of the dominant notions of taste, Lady Gaga's personal experience of (albeit temporary) disability provides an important opportunity to revisit her previous use of disability imagery, particularly within the context of high versus pop culture and her embrace of subjugated 'monsters'.

Uptight About Difference?

When Lady Gaga appeared as a mermaid and used a wheelchair during a Sydney performance in 2011, she was again met with criticism from a number of sectors, including the disability blogosphere, spinal cord research centres, Madonna fans and the Divine Miss M – Bette Midler herself. As two postings show:

Dear @ladygaga how about using your celebrity status 2 try 2 get us out of wheelchairs instead of cruising one. Cool?! @spinalcordcure (Roman Reed Foundation, 2011)

Since this isn't the first time she has used a wheelchair in her performances, I invite her to learn more about the 5.6 million Americans who live with paralysis … They, like me, unfortunately, don't use a wheelchair for shock value. (Grossberg, 2011)

These two critiques illustrate different ways of understanding disability. Firstly, the tweet from the Roman Reed Foundation, a spinal cord research centre, illustrates the medical model of disability which sees disability as a problem within an individual's body which should be cured. The second comment, from a wheelchair user, illustrates the social model of disability which posits that people's attitudes are disabling and result in social exclusion from the workforce and other aspects of ordinary community life. Neither critique, however, celebrates the inclusion of disability within popular culture or recognises the ongoing position of disability and the image of the wheelchair in popular music moments of cultural critique. According to Gagapedia, Lady

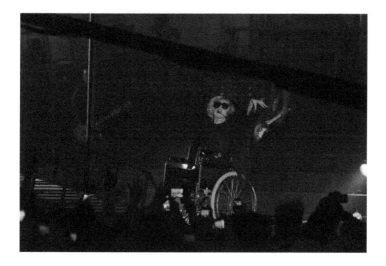

Figure 6.1   Lady Gaga appears onstage as Yuyi the mermaid at 2011 Sydney Concert

Source: © Danielle Smith/Fairfax Syndication.

Gaga used the wheelchair to 'keep herself "mobile" on stage since she wore a mermaid tail' (Gagapedia, no date).

This disability imagery is an experimentation with what has come before. Lady Gaga is not the first non-disabled performer to appropriate the wheelchair as a symbol of disability to make some kind of cultural critique. In 1978 Bette Midler also appeared onstage in a wheelchair and dressed as a mermaid, while in 1992 Kurt Cobain wheeled around the stage in a wheelchair while wearing a blonde wig and hospital gown at the Reading Festival. Cobain's performance, which was reported as a 'comment on media speculations about his mental health' (Cook, 2013) and would indeed be his last UK show, was referenced in 2013 at the same festival when the English folk/punk singer-songwriter Frank Turner, having recently sustained a back injury, appeared onstage in a wheelchair rather than cancel the gig. His explanation that the appearance was an ode to Cobain was met with criticism from disability rights groups.

Midler, who perhaps inspired all of these performances, including Cobain's, offered a light hearted critique of the reference within Lady Gaga's broader persona:

> Dear @ladygaga Ive been doing singing mermaid in a wheelchair since 1980- You can keep the meat dress and the firecracker tits-mermaid's mine. (Midler cited in Casablanca and Weisman, 2011)

With the exception of (possibly) Turner, none of these performers actually required a wheelchair; however, the presence of the wheelchair is itself a significant image. For example, when Robert Wyatt performed *I'm a Believer* on *Top of the Pops* in 1974 following his paralysis, the producers of the show, afraid about how a wheelchair would be received, attempted to hide its presence through tight camera framing and by covering his legs with a blanket (G. McKay, 2013, p. 104). McKay also discusses the way talented, yet obviously disabled, musicians such as Kata Kolbert never gained popular success because 'we do not want female pop singers in wheelchairs' (p. 90), and further considers the tendency for the popular music press to predict the end of careers when musicians such as the talented 1970s soul singer Teddy Pendergrass became wheelchair users (p. 96).

However, at least two key Australian cultural commentators with disabilities responded positively to Lady Gaga's Sydney wheelchair performance. Celebrity blogger and media personality Stella Young noted that it was logical that a mermaid would require a mobility aid and suggested that the most vocal critiques came from the perspective that disability should be cured, not alleviated with accessible environments:

> But Gaga isn't telling a story about disability. She's not portraying or mimicking people with disabilities. I don't really think she's even making a statement about disability, and if she is, it's not a negative one. If she's sending the message that a wheelchair is a liberating solution to a mobility impairment, whether it's a disability or a big black vinyl mermaid tail, I reckon that serves us wheelchair users pretty well. (Young, 2011)

Young uses Lady Gaga's wheelchair performance as an opportunity to advocate for social justice and adequate support for people with disability as opposed to campaigning for a cure. This argument has previously found traction within the popular music arena when Teddy Pendergrass distanced himself from Christopher Reeve's campaign to cure spinal cord injury, preferring instead to use his pop profile for social change to emphasise 'quality of life' (Pendergrass cited in G. McKay, 2013, p. 101).

The other commentator, Griffith University activist academic Fiona Kumari Campbell, describes the critiques of Lady Gaga as evidence of a moral indignation in society regarding disability. Kumari Campbell interrogates the negative reaction to Lady Gaga's embrace of disability imagery in her Sydney concert:

> My concern about this whole media drama is the deployment of moral righteousness when it comes to disability. Is disability so awful that the public is forced to remain in a state of permanent uptightness – to enact a fabrication

where disability is everywhere but daily erasure provokes invisibility? Again, the issue of who has the right to speak on behalf of disabled people arises. What I love about the Gaga show is that disability has presence in the same way she refers of the other forms of marginality – ability discrimination (or ableism as I refer to it) even sneaks into the lyrics of her hit anthem "Born This Way". (Campbell, 2011)

Kumari Campbell raises an important point about the daily erasure invoking invisibility. Whereas disability theorists often describe disability as being 'everywhere' but unfortunately written out of culture, the music industry has tended to obscure the presence of disability, unless it is used as a specific marketing strategy. For example, Lady Gaga, who invokes disability themes in her creation of a pop persona, has been heavily criticised in the disability blogosphere for her appropriation of the image of disability in a form of 'crip drag' or exploitation of the disabled (Hamilton, 2009).

Popular Culture is the Culture that People Deem Relevant to Their Lives

With Lady Gaga curating a legion of little monster followers, a number of her fans have posted performances of her music on YouTube. This is especially important for people with disabilities who, as Cameron (2009) argues, have had limited access to the means of producing cultural resources. With the advent of web 2.0 and YouTube in particular, large numbers of people with disabilities have become cultural producers, using Lady Gaga music to create their own videos. For example deaf communities have used online platforms to create sign language translations of her music. *Born this Way* in particular has emerged on YouTube as an anthem for the disability rights agenda, with both individuals with disabilities and flash mob groups of people with disabilities uploading their performances of the song which includes lyrics such as:

Don't hide yourself in regret
Just love yourself and you're set
I'm on the right track, baby
I was born this way, born this way

Although the song may not explicitly be about disability, its message of inclusion and being happy with who you are has become part of the popular culture of people with disabilities who have turned to YouTube in a kind of cultural bricolage. Fiske (1989, 2010) acknowledges that while the practice of compiling your own album (writing in the 1980s, he referred to mix tapes) may not be ideologically resistive, it allows subordinated groups to 'make their own culture' in a way that transforms 'readers into cultural producers, not consumers' (p. 119).

Conclusion

Several disability music theorists note the absence of disability theorisation within music studies and argue that both disciplines could gain much insight from the other (Cain, 2010; Lerner and Straus, 2006; Straus, 2011). Joseph Straus' *Extraordinary Measures: Disability in Music* is one of the few investigations of the intersections between disability and music. However, it is necessarily limited to exclude popular music for theoretical and practical reasons. George McKay (2013) takes many of the insights raised in these earlier explorations of largely classical music and applies them to popular music in *Shakin' All Over: Popular Music and Disability* in an attempt to contribute to a cultural investigation of the images of disability that influence our understanding of human difference (p. 190). This chapter took popular music and Lady Gaga as its case study to attempt a similar investigation of the importance of disability in popular music's counterculture of otherness.

Lady Gaga occupies a position of both otherness and mass appeal (Corona, 2011). She appeals to many people and situates herself, through her embrace of otherness, as being of the people (Fiske, 1986). She is popular culture. Her appropriation of images of the disabled demonstrates a knowledge of and innovation with formulas of popular culture. Whereas some have taken literal interpretations of her use of disability images as damaging to the disabled who are trying to establish themselves as ordinary people with ordinary problems (Gray, 2012; Grossberg, 2011; Hamilton, 2009), others recognise the political potential of an inclusion of disability within the glamor that surrounds the pop star (Dilling-Hansen, 2012). This chapter reads Lady Gaga's use of disability imagery as an act of both consumption and production, to offer an analysis of Lady Gaga's popular culture as a political representation of disability. These politics also encompass the critiques she has prompted.

While Lady Gaga is a significant contemporary example due to her appropriation of and experimentation with historic formulations of popular culture as well as her willingness to embrace difference, disability has occupied a central position throughout pop music history through performers such as Ian Dury, Johnny Rotten and Ian Curtis and the industry's general fascination with otherness.

Chapter 7

Controlling the Body: Sport, Disability and the Construction of Ability

Muhammad Ali and Floyd Mayweather are world champion boxers. However, had they been engaged in the sport during the same era, they would never have competed against each other. Boxing is divided into classes so that athletes of different weights, heights and ability can compete against each other fairly. Whereas Ali was a heavyweight boxer, Mayweather competes in a range of lighter weight classes. The elite disability sports event the Paralympics similarly operates under a classification system where people with different impairments are grouped into competing classes. While boxing divisions are rarely criticised as too complicated or detrimental to the viewing experience, broadcasters are fearful that similar systems in disability sports alienate audiences.

Sport is an important element of popular culture that brings together a number of symbolic forces and stereotypes, including heroes, icons, rituals and clearly defined social roles. This chapter interrogates these seemingly spontaneous events and roles to consider the careful orchestration of meaning they contain. For example, the supercrip often emerges in disability sports as a stereotype that governs the way people construct themselves and others. As Silva and Howe (2012) explain, 'the tendency for disability supercripization [in disability sports] may be amplified to serve interests that might not be aligned with ideals of empowerment' (p. 181).

The global sport industry expanded throughout the twentieth century and became increasingly commercialised (Rowe, 1995, p. 101), an aspect that continues into this century. While some criticise this commercialisation of sport as having a corrupting influence, of destroying sport's essential being and its true aesthetic beauty, others argue that sport provides people from marginalised groups the opportunity to participate and excel. Following Toby Miller (2001), this chapter recognises the importance of this commercialisation, to argue that sport, and sport advertising, represents a highly commoditised arena in which we can analyse the politics of social change. Whereas Miller focused on race, gender and sexuality, similar changes are evident in disability sports, and particularly the Paralympics. However, these changes, evident through the increasing commodification of particular sports celebrities, should not be celebrated unproblematically because a 'behind-the-scenes' inequality continues to exist (Miller, 2001, p. 10). However, in this chapter I will argue that, in the case of disability, inequality is not necessarily behind-the-scenes.

The chapter begins with a discussion of sport as popular culture and the contradictions and ambiguities this form of entertainment and physical pursuit opens up, before moving on to outline a brief history of the Paralympic games as it emerged in Britain through a rehabilitative discourse following the Second World War. The chapter then turns to a consideration of the way ability is accommodated in disabled sports, being wary of the continued discourse of the supercrip that pervades this arena. In recognition that sport has, in many ways, turned into a media and commercial event, this chapter draws case studies from media representations of disabled sports – including shifting discourses around Oscar Pistorius, the *Meet the Superhumans* campaign, successive coverage of Paralympic games and the successful documentary film *Murderball* – to interrogate the cultural construction of ability.

Disability, Sport and Popular Culture

While talent and disability seem to be cultural opposites, both disability and super-ability (or athleticism) can be viewed as deviations from 'the norm' (van Hilvoorde and Landeweerd, 2008). This concept is again foundational to critical disability studies, as Kim Q. Hall (2011) illustrates with the example of Caster Semenya and the controversy surrounding her gender during the 2009 Olympic games. Hall explains that Semenya, who was precluded from competition and forced to undergo gender verification testing, has an extraordinary body, just as people marked disabled do.

Sport is a complicated example of popular culture that draws influence from changing technology, everyday life, commercialisation, entertainment, beauty and aesthetics. The connection between disability and competitive sport may seem paradoxical because, in order to excel at sport, the athlete must be extraordinarily talented, or significantly more *able* than the general population, and indeed the other athletes against whom they are competing. However, Umberto Eco's observations about the athlete resonates within disability studies as examples of extraordinary bodies:

> The athlete is already a being who has hypertroplized one organ, who turns his body into the seat and exclusive source of a continuous play. The athlete is a monster, he is The Man Who Laughs, the geisha with the compressed and atrophied foot, dedicated to total instrumentalication. (Eco, 1987 [1969, cited in Miller p. 2])

The athlete's body is different, associated with the abnormal, and used for the purposes of our entertainment. Like the circus freak, the athlete elicits amazement – the 'wow climax' Jenkins describes. However, unlike the freak, the athlete also provokes feelings of admiration and respect. Indeed, an important cultural distinction occurs at the moment 'amazement ... turn[s] into admiration when an "extraordinary feature" is mastered and turns out to be an extraordinary sport talent' (van Hilvoorde and Landeweerd, 2008, p. 104). As academic and ex-paralympian Danielle Peers (2009) explains, the media representation and public's perception of disability sports continue to be influenced by somewhat opposing discourses of the nineteenth-century freak show, rehabilitation and mainstream sport. However, where the athlete is culturally revered, the person with disability is not. Yet disability pervades sport and, as Eco's observations cited above attest, impairment and injury mark the athlete's body as badges of honour and evidence of true dedication to the subculture (Miller, 2001).

According to Rosemarie Garland-Thomson, extraordinary bodies provide the boundary by which the normate is defined. The normate is 'the figure outlined by an array of deviant others whose marked bodies shore up the norm's boundaries ... [It] is the constructed identity of those who, by way of the bodily configurations and cultural capital they assume, can step into a position of authority and wield the power it grants them' (Garland-Thomson 1997 cited in K.Q. Hall, 2011, p. 3). So, while Hilvoorde and Landwaeerd argue that the athlete has an extraordinary body, Kim Q. Hall expands on this, identifying that, even within this extraordinary system, a hierarchy exists between acceptable and unacceptable bodies. Such observations shed light on the construction and maintenance of ability. For example, Susan Wendell describes the belief that it is possible to have the body we desire – the 'myth of control' – yet identifies its insidious cultural maintenance:

> There are other popular versions of the myth of control. One is the belief that if you take proper care of your body, you will stay fit and well until you die (presumably death will be instantaneous and inexplicable). This has the ugly implication that if you are ill or disabled, you must have failed to take care of yourself. (Wendell, 1996, p. 103)

The myth of control pervades wheelchair sports. In a study of five male and four female wheelchair athletes, Kim Wickman (2007) found that 'the discourse of able-ism has considerable impact on the way the athletes understand themselves and the world, and, thus, on their identity construction' (p. 151). During interviews the wheelchair athletes sought to emphasise their ability and sporting dominance. They sought in particular to differentiate themselves from 'others' whom they saw as having very severe impairments.

Fiona Kumari Campbell (2009) suggests an investigation of ableism as the next step in rethinking not only disability, but 'all bodies and mentalities within the parameters of nature/culture' (p. 198). Several cultural disability theorists offer a framework for this interrogation by identifying the discursive function of disability. They offer definitions of 'disability' which reveal its role in shoring up concepts of 'ability':

> … the real limitation from which they must escape. (Mitchell and Snyder, 2000, p. 2)

> …. the other that helps make otherness imaginable. (Siebers 2008, p. 48)

> … a system for interpreting and disciplining bodily variations. (Garland-Thomson, 2011, p. 17)

These theorists seek to understand how disability functions as an identity category and a category of deviance which helps to shore up its opposite – ability – which they argue is a cultural construction designed to make people feel more secure in their tenuous bodies.

In the vein of examining whiteness as a concept within critical race theory or masculinity within gender studies, Fiona Kumari Campbell suggests we should 'shift our gaze and concentrate on what the study of disability tells us about the production, operation and maintenance of ableism' (2009, p. 4). Kumari Campbell situates ableism as a cultural project that is repeatedly performed and difficult to sustain because, by their very nature, all bodies are out of control – people with disability are an acute reminder of the temporariness of an able-bodied ontology. As these critical disability theorists argue, the binary between us/them and able/disabled is not easy to maintain.

Cultural theorist Stuart Hall (1997) argues that social- and stereo-types occur in moments of social inequality. The dominant group attempts to establish a concept of normality that, through repetition, appears naturalised, almost automatic. Representation is crucial to this process because of the role it plays in the construction of identity. For example, the supercrip, a disability stereotype referred to throughout this book, is a clearly defined role for the disabled athlete that is repeatedly represented and performed to the point that it has become 'common sense'. For example, Danielle Peers explores the insidious nature of the Paralympic narrative in the media discourses surrounding her own career:

> I read the newspaper articles and press releases that others have written about me. I read my own grant applications, speeches and business cards. I read myself defined, in each of these, by one word: not crip, queer, athlete, activist, student, woman or lesbian, but Paralympian. I read my entire life story transformed into

that of The Paralympian. I see my origins declared, not at the moment of my birth, but at some tragic moment of my physical disablement. I read my new coherent life narrative: my salvation from the depths of my disability by the progressive, benevolent empowerment of sport. My destiny reads as a coming of age. I am the heroic Paralympian: pedestal, medal and all. (Peers, 2009, p. 654)

She goes on to outline the way this discourse afforded her inclusion, yet at a broader social cost, 'I see how it renders me anonymous, just as it renders me famous. I feel how it renders me passive, so that it can empower me' (Peers, 2009, p. 654). Peers thus questions the discourse of 'empowerment' that surround the supercripisation of Paralympians arguing that such a characterisation in fact perpetuates a culturally enforced passivity and marginal status of people with disability.

History of the Paralympics

Although people with disability have been participating in sport and sports clubs since the 1800s – and in a variety of sports from pole dancing to body building – the Paralympics is the most widely known disabled sports event in popular culture. Through these games we can see a gradual shifting focus in disability sports from rehabilitation to recreation, to recently where disabled athletes have been recognised as on par with elite athletes. The 2012 Paralympic games was integral in raising the profile of disability sports and shifting the focus from rehabilitation to elite sporting ability.

The history of the Paralympics games began at Stoke Mandeville Hospital in the UK following the Second World War where participation in sport was a compulsory aspect of rehabilitation. Neurologist Sir Ludwig Guttmann believed in the rehabilitative potential of sport in:

... restoring the disabled person's physical fitness i.e.: his (sic) strength, coordination, speed and endurance ... restoring that passion for playful activity and the desire to experience joy and pleasure in life ... promoting that psychological equilibrium which enables the disabled to come to terms with his physical defect, to develop activity of mind, self confidence, self dignity, self discipline, competitive spirit, and comradeship, mental attitudes ... to facilitate and accelerate his social re-integration and integration. (Guttmann 1976 cited in Thomas, 2008, p. 26)

Guttmann sought to encourage people with spinal cord injury and those disabled during the war to participate in sport as a means of rehabilitation, and organised the Stoke Mandeville games in 1948 to coincide with the

Olympic games being held in London the same year. Twenty-six British veterans, including three women, competed in wheelchair archery at these games (DePauw and Gavron, 2005). Guttmann selected archery because of its rehabilitative and integrative potential. He maintained that it was 'of immense value in strengthening, in a very natural way, just those muscles of the upper limbs, shoulders and trunk, on which the paraplegic's well-balanced, upright position depends' (Guttmann 1952 cited in Brittain, 2013). Following the games, a number of athletes joined local archery clubs.

Throughout the 1960s the games developed into an international sporting event that took place every 4 years. Whereas in 1960, 23 countries took part, in 2012 164 did. Although Guttmann has been remembered as single-minded in his focus on people with spinal cord injuries (Thomas, 2008), the Stoke Mandeville games eventually opened to people with other physical and visual impairments in 1976.

The competition came to be known as the Paralympics in 1984. Athletes with disability are now categorised according to the following categories:

> Wheelchair athletes; athletes with cerebral palsy; amputees; athletes with total or partial loss of sight; athletes with learning disability and learning difficulties; "les autres" disabilities (a complex "all the rest category"). (van Hilvoorde and Landeweerd, 2008, pp. 98–9)

Various bodies have overseen the development of disability sports as it has transitioned from a medicalised categorisation to functional classification system. The earlier medical 'class-based' classification meant that only people with the same impairment could compete against each other, for example an athlete with a paraplegic spinal cord injury and a double above-knee amputee could not compete against each other in a wheelchair race. However, as the rules shifted to recognise that people with different impairments had the same or similar level of function, the games became more focused on sport. The International Paralympic Committee (IPC) describe the purpose of functional classification as an equalising measure designed to 'minimize the impact of impairment on the outcome of competition' (IPC, 2014). This process is often described as 'levelling the playing field'.

Classification

Peter van der Vliet, Chief Medical Officer for the IPC, describes classification as the relationship between impairment and sporting activity and outlines the way athletes are awarded a number of points based on the advantages and disadvantages their impairment poses in relation to the specific sport:

In swimming, for instance, many will wonder how a dwarf can compete against a paraplegic. Swimming is a complex discipline and in Paralympic terms, it's not purely about getting from A to B. It also involves the complexities of a start, turning point, stroke length, stroke rate, buoyancy, and frontal drag. (Vliet, 2012)

While the Olympics only have one men's 100m finals, the functional classification system means that the Paralympics has 14. However, as mentioned previously, this is not unique to disability sports – some able-bodied sports such as boxing and judo adopt similar classification schemes related to age, weight or height. Athletes compete in 'classes', or, as in the case of wheelchair rugby, a number of points are awarded to each member of the team and the team as a whole is allowed a maximum number of points on the field at any one time.

The Paralympic movement now attempts a comprehensive approach to the classification of impairment and resulting inclusion of athletes as influenced by the World Health Organization. The games consist of a number of different sports, each with their own specific rules. Some are disability-specific, some are not. To summarise:

Each Paralympic Sport has to clearly define for which impairment groups they provide sports opportunities. This is described in the Classification Rules of each sport. While some sports include athletes of all impairment types (e.g. Athletics, Swimming), other sports are limited to one impairment type (e.g. Goalball, Boccia) or a selection of impairment types (e.g. Equestrian, Cycling). The presence of an applicable eligible impairment is a prerequisite but not the sole criterion of entry into a particular Paralympic Sport. (IPC, 2014)

For example, in blind soccer, accommodations are made to equalise different levels of vision loss and specific positions allow for sighted players:

There are five players on each team and the game lasts 50 minutes. Rules are similar to the able-bodied game with a few modifications. The ball makes noise when it moves and everyone, aside from the goalkeeper, uses eye shades to ensure fairness. The goalkeeper may be sighted and act as a guide during the game. Also, the measurements on the field are smaller and there are no offside rulings. (International Paralympic Committee (IPC) n.d)

Despite audiences and broadcasters criticising the functional classification system for being too complicated to understand, the focus on function and altering the environment to allow people to compete on an equal level is an important tenant of social oppression models of disability. Through the points and classification systems, the Paralympics attempt to remove barriers to full participation. However, some athletes with disability do seek to compete against their able-bodied peers, and such examples will be discussed below.

Inclusion

When Oscar Pistorius, an amputee who runs with J-shaped carbon fibre prosthetics, sought to compete against non-disabled athletes at the 2008 Olympics, the International Association of Athletics Federations (IAAF) amended competition rules to exclude the use of 'any technical device that incorporates springs, wheels, or any other such element that provides a user with an advantage over another athlete not using such a device' (IAAF Rule 144.2 cited in van Hilvoorde and Landeweerd, 2008, p. 106). A spokesperson for the IAAF claimed the committee was ruling in anticipation of the development of future technology and held nothing against Pistorius specifically (Nick Davis cited in van Hilvoorde and Landeweerd, 2008). Although the decision was eventually overturned and Pistorius did not place in his qualifying race, the debate raised a number of intriguing questions about disability, sport, extra-ability and technology. If, as the IAAF argued, Pistorius had an unfair advantage over able-bodied athletes, what kind of advantage did he have over the disabled athletes against whom he had been competing for years (Swartz and Watermeyer, 2008)?

Pistorius thus emerged as an 'ambiguous figure' in debates regarding deficit models of disability, the merging of humans and technology, the commercialisation of sport, and unfair advantage in sport (Burkett, McNamee, and Potthast, 2011). Although Pistorius was not able to compete at the 2008 games, he opened a debate about sport, the limits of the human body, and if prosthetics posed an advantage over the natural body. Since then Pistorius has gone on to receive gold at the 2011 World Championships in athletics and competed in the 400m relay at the 2012 Olympic games.

However, as this book goes to print he has been found guilty of the manslaughter of his girlfriend Reeva Steenkamp, jeopardising any near-future sporting endeavours.

However, it must be noted that Pistorius was not the first disabled athlete to compete at the Olympics. In 1904, George Eyser competed in gymnastics on a wooden leg and won three gold medals. Neroli Hairhall a paraplegic archer, competed at the 1984 games, while Marla Runyan was a blind runner who competed in the 1500m athletics competition in 2000 at the Sydney Olympics (van Hilvoorde and Landeweerd, 2008).

To conclude, despite disability sports first appearing as exhibition events at the Olympic games in 1984, the inclusion of disabled athletes remains controversial. Such an inclusion blurs the boundary separating able and disabled. However, Pistorius' prosthetics also reveal the way people with disability rely on

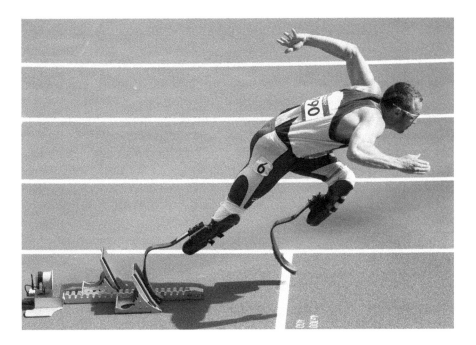

Figure 7.1   Oscar Pistorius competes in the Men's 400m Round 1 Heats on Day 8 of the London 2012 Olympic Games at the Olympic Stadium on August 4, 2012 in London

Source: © Getty Images.

technology to participate in everyday life and sport. Although disabled sports recognise difference, divisions continue to be created through the cultural and media maintenance of a normative body.

The Media Love an Inspiration

Silva and Howe (2012) describe the Paralympics as a potentially transgressive global event but caution that 'the increasing media influence and economic importance of the Paralympics means ... we should pay careful attention to the modes of representation disseminated and their possible implications' (p. 181). Throughout this book I have considered the ways commercialised mass culture is turned into popular culture and highlighted the importance of messages of resistance that emerge, are poached or interpreted, despite popular culture's relationship with commercialisation. In the context of disability sports as popular culture, this is especially significant.

In *Playing on the Periphery*, Tara Brabazon (2006) argues that sport as an object of popular culture is not 'an isolated social and political formation' (p. 2). She uses sport to counter the view that popular culture is trash and suggests instead that popular culture can be interrogated for its aesthetic values, embrace and reflection of technological change and its reflections of political conflict, everyday life and economics. Brabazon's analysis of sport as popular culture dependent on aesthetics, technology, the quotidian and economics is evident in the discourses surrounding Oscar Pistorius. Prior to shooting his girlfriend in 2013, Pistorius was *the face* of disability and sport and was often held up as an image of inspiration and of the fruits of strong will and determination. Blind adventurer and motivational speaker Erik Weihenmayer's 2008 description of the athlete became a popular internet meme which, as I discuss in the next chapter, prompted the creation of a disability- and internet-specific literary critique of the supercrip. The below quote accompanied an image of Pistorius poised to race wearing his famous 'blade runner' prosthetic legs:

> Through birth or circumstance some are given certain gifts. But it's what one does with those gifts, the hours devoted to training, the desire to be the best that is at the true heart of a champion. (Weihenmayer, 2008)

An image of both disability and extreme strength, Pistorius was a high powered commodity when he sought to compete against able-bodied competitors at the Olympic games in 2008. As I discuss in the following chapter, these inspirational images are not intended to promote the social inclusion of people with disability, they work instead to reassure the non-disabled that at least there is someone in a worse situation than themselves. Australian disability blogger Stella Young attributes the Pistorius images to a cultural phenomenon she described as 'inspiration porn' (Young, 2012).

Since Steenkamp's death, Pistorius has become an even more ambiguous figure. No longer a high-powered commodity, he was dropped by his sponsor Nike overnight. Pistorius has transitioned from the inspirational supercrip to the disabled supervillain right before our eyes. This can be seen most clearly in the changing media frames applied to this sporting figure (see Ellis and Goggin, 2015).

Lack of Media Interest

In addition to the repetitive inspirational supercrip media frames, the Paralympics has also suffered from an absence of media interest. A comparative analysis of Olympics and Paralympics newspaper coverage conducted during the 2000 Sydney and 2002 Salt Lake City games discovered that 'the Paralympics received approximately 2.7 per cent of the coverage of the Olympics' (Bertling and Schierl, 2008, p. 43). In addition to this stark quantitative difference, qualitative differences emerged around what was reported. To return to Peers' observations around the construction of the 'Paralympic narrative', she recounts the media's disregard for the 1996 Atlanta Paralympic games:

> After the Olympics closed, the media left, they took down all the signs, the cafeteria did not have enough food, there was no toilet paper for the athletes to use – they just gutted the space and left the Paralympic athletes to fend for themselves. (Peers cited in Alary, 2012)

Schell and Duncan (1999) argue that in CBS's coverage of these games, commentators often implied competitors should simply be 'grateful for the Paralympic experience' (p. 35). They describe this as patronising and a process of othering. Othering reduces the complexity of a situation or experience to a single characteristic. While Thomas and Smith (2003) attribute the disregard for Paralympic sports to a certain degree on its rehabilitative origins, media descriptions of elite athletes with disabilities usually invoke medical terminology that locates the cause for disability in the body. Further, the discourse of disability criticism has not been able to articulate a mode of critique that recognises the relationship disability and ability have with history. Channel 4, the UK broadcasters of the 2012 London Paralympics, made a concerted effort to reverse this media discourse through a comprehensive marketing campaign designed to attract an audience. They embarked on an unapologetically commercial approach to integrating disability into sporting entertainment and aesthetics.

Attracting an Audience

Popular sport is a media event that relies on attracting an audience. Competitive sports media attempt to leverage an audience by including 'additional information, aesthetic or emotional in nature, which allows a particular sport to offer its audience more than mere athletic action' (Bertling and Schierl, 2008, p. 41). While Paralympic athletes have backstories which offer these extra details, they may not be viewed as purely entertaining and could in fact elicit discomfort rather than aesthetic appreciation. As the broader media representation of sport becomes increasingly commercialised and journalists and audiences seek out 'light entertainment', disability sports become harder to sell because of the social issues attached to disability. In addition, the disabled athlete's body is not seen as aesthetically pleasing and disability sports itself does not fit into the category of 'pure entertainment' Yet, the Paralympics relies on the media to increase interest in the event (Bertling and Schierl, 2008, p. 41).

While interest in the Paralympics has dramatically improved since the IPC partnered with the International Olympics Committee (IOC) and brokered sponsorship deals with multinational corporations such as VISA and Johnson and Johnson, corporate sponsorship was recently described as the 'the largest gap in equitable treatment' between Paralympic and Olympic athletes during the Sochi Paralympics (CBCNews.Ca, 2014). However, the requirement that the Olympics' host nation similarly agree to host the Paralympics has also seen interest improve. Despite this, media coverage has remained, at times, problematic.

Because it was not seen as a profitable, marketable event, the Paralympics has not previously gained much media attention. However, television rights for the 2012 event were sold on the open market in the UK for the first time. Channel 4 successfully bid £8 million and embarked on a new era of disability sports, hoping to 'bring about a fundamental shift in perceptions of disability in the UK' (Channel 4 Press, 2010). Their specific aims were to:

Position the London 2012 Paralympic Games as one of the largest broadcast events of 2012 and the biggest event in Channel 4's history
Engage the UK media early and move coverage for Paralympic sport from the margins to the mainstream
Prepare the ground for the biggest, loudest marketing campaign in the Channel's history (*Thanks for the Warm Up* and *Meet the Superhumans*)
Sustain momentum from the Olympics and direct public interest towards Channel 4's Paralympic coverage
Reinforce Channel 4's long-standing identity as an innovator prepared to challenge perceptions, break new boundaries and provide a voice for the minority audience
Bring about a shift in public attitudes to disability. (CIPR, 2012)

Channel 4 adopted a comprehensive PR strategy in their attempt to move the Paralympics from the margins of media attention to the mainstream. Perhaps the more significant move was simply treating the Paralympic games as a significant sporting event. Indeed, unlike the situation Peers recounted at the 1996 games where the media left, in 2012 the Olympics were used as a transitional PR measure to elicit interest in the Paralympics.

Table 7.1 outlines Channel 4's marketing and broadcast strategy as it focused on education, excitement, anticipation and reputation over a 2-year period. The strategy reflects the argument that sport as popular culture involves a complex mix of aesthetics, technology, economics and the everyday. In their attempt to make the Paralympics a commercial event with an audience attached, Channel 4 embarked on reshaping the disabled athletic aesthetic into an image that invoked feeling of amazement *and* admiration. New technological systems were also employed to ensure audience comprehension and interest. The LEXI decoder system was designed to 'unlock' the classification system by illustrating onscreen through coloured graphics the different levels of impairment in each class. Economically, a number of key stakeholders were involved as were different industries from PR to research and evaluation. Channel 4 engaged sports communications agency Pitch to give the Paralympics a reputation overhaul and create an entirely new audience. An advertisement of the UK Paralympic team called *Meet the Superhumans* was key to their onslaught and has initiated a new aesthetic in sports celebrity and advertising.

Table 7.1   Channel 4 2012 Paralympics Marketing Strategy

Strategy	Date	Features
Education	2010–2012	Engage PR specialists Develop cross-promotional opportunities with Paralympic editorial team at C4 Launch £500k initiative to search for new disabled Paralympic presenters Begin publicity for Paralympic programming
Excitement	January 2012–July 2012	Announce line up of disabled talent LEXI decoder system announced Roadshow to offices of key TV listing, consumer and feature media Commission bespoke photography of athletes and presenters Prepare comprehensive crisis comms plan with buy in from key stakeholders (including LOCOG, IPC and BPA)
Anticipation	July/August 2012	*Meet the Superhumans* campaign launch Roll out C4 presenters, athletes and executives Hold one-to-one briefings with each national sports editors Lobby TV listings media against drop-off of coverage after the Olympics Build profile of LEXI decoder system and Paralympics presenters through 'paid for' supplements in key nationals and regionals papers
Reputation	During and post-games	Place presenter columns in broadsheet press Commission research Host journalists and celebrations at the games

The Superhumans: A New Aesthetics of Bodily Imperfection?

Meet the Superhumans, the edgy ad featuring Paralympians as athletes to be admired for their strength, speed and physical agility, was designed to create a mass audience for the games and change public perceptions about disability. The ad went viral after being released on YouTube. The athletic triumphs of the athletes are interspersed with scenes such as a pregnant woman pacing a hospital hallway, a soldier being blown up and a horrific car accident, all set to an adrenalin-pumping soundtrack – Public Enemy's *Harder Than You Think*. These traditionally framed tragic moments are hailed through the paradigm shifting soundtrack as defining moments in the creation of strong, competitive athletes. Dan Brookes, the creator of the campaign, describes the ad as replacing the 'ahh bless' perceptions of people with disability competing in the Paralympic games with a 'cool factor'. Brooke's goal was to create 'something bold, awe-inspiring and unapologetic to capture the public's imagination' (Scope, 2012).

Meet the Superhumans has been described as reversing attitudes that Paralympic athletes are objects of pity. Compare the images featured in this ad with the observations of this Paralympic athlete competing in the 1984 games:

> The BBC has a 45-minute programme on them and it was very … I was going to say derogatory, derisive, but they were just demeaning really … In an "oh look at these disabled people, aren't they marvellous …. Getting out there and doing something" …. Patronising, I think, is probably the best description. (Thomas, 2008, p. 138)

This athlete did not see successive coverage in Seoul or Sydney as much better. While *Meet the Superhumans* still focused on the backstory of the athletes, it did not frame tragedy as the main feature of the story. Evaluation of the campaign suggests it did successfully change attitudes towards disability sports, but whether it changed attitudes to disability more generally is another question. *Meet the Superhumans* has won a number of awards and Channel 4 was awarded the broadcast rights to the 2014 and 2016 games on the back of their 2012 broadcast. The success of the marketing campaign and coverage of the games can be demonstrated by successive surveys finding more Britains could name a Paralympian following the games in 2012 than back in 2010 (18–41%) when first surveyed (Media Centre, 2012). While this research shows us that an audience can be created for disability sports where one previously didn't exist, the questions remains as to the impact the games actually had on changing public perceptions of disability, especially within the context of welfare reforms currently underway.

Disability Now columnist Peter White compares the support received by Paralympian Jonnie Peacock to the experiences of a woman attempting to appeal the decision that she is fit for work and so should have her benefits cut. White argues that the adulation afforded to the Paralympic athletes does not equate to understanding:

Peacock, Weir, Simmonds and many of the others are super athletes. Admiring and recognising their talent is great, but it contributes about as much to an understanding of disability as cheering on Mo Farah contributes to understanding Somalians and welcoming them to this country. It's oranges and apples, and even expecting it to happen was painfully naive. (White, 2013)

White's critique is in stark contrast to the largely celebratory analysis of Channel 4's coverage of the games and the award winning Superhuman campaign:

Channel4 changed perceptions of disability in the UK, attracted a record-breaking audience, affirmed its public service remit and succeeded in delivering a commercial return. The positive reception to our bid to broadcast Rio 2016 is further evidence of ROI for delivering successfully on our PR objectives. (CIPR, 2012)

However, disability commentators, including some athletes have used the intense media and public interest now surrounding the Paralympics to highlight important disability social justice issues such as the impacts austerity measures will have on the next generation of Paralympic athletes who may have to make difficult decisions regarding what to spend their money on. Similarly, both Channel 4 and the Paralympics were targeted by protestors because one of the sponsors of the Games –ATOS – had also been contracted by the Department for Work and Pensions to carry out the controversial 'fitness to work' tests.

Indeed, it is interesting to note that the celebrated Superhumans campaign describes the athletes as superhuman – a word Clogston specifically listed within the supercrip (traditional) frame of news coverage of disability, discussed in Chapter 3. Does this campaign differ from other traditional frames of disability because the people with disabilities portrayed as superhuman within the *Meet the Superhuman* campaign are superhuman *because of* their athleticism not *in spite of* their disability?

Sport, and particularly the Olympics, is a site of popular culture where feelings of national pride are elicited and performed. This has not been the case for the Paralympics where athletes are characterised as individuals overcoming adversary rather than representatives of a nation, as this wheelchair athlete explains:

It is as if people cannot identify with a disabled person. I mean, when Sweden wins a gold medal in archery (...) or ice hockey or football or pentathlon or something – then it is "we" who win the gold medal. If it is a disabled person who wins a gold medal – then it is "they". It is not "We – Sweden". (Wickman, 2007, p.157)

Meet the Superhumans draws on the aesthetics of the athlete in the context of disability to change this. Drawing on Hans Ulrich, Gumbrecht argues that the aesthetic appeal of the athlete's perfect body provides a vital means of escapism, Bertling and Schierl (2008) believe the disabled athlete competing in the Paralympics games can be 'treated aesthetically by the media' (p. 49). *Meet the Superhumans* has clear aesthetic value and entertainment aspects. Unlike a lot of other Paralympic coverage which either obscures impairment or focuses on results, *Meet the Superhumans* embraces the 'pure' entertainment aspect of the Paralympics.

Advertising the Athletic Aesthetic – 'With it' Compulsory Able-Bodiedness?

The aesthetic has been replicated by the Canadian Winter Paralympics with their *It's Not What's Missing* advertisement (see Laird, 2014). Similarly, Duracell's *Trust Your Power* advertisement, which features hearing impaired footballer Derrick Coleman, adopts the same strategy of aligning disability, masculinity and athleticism with a cool factor never before applied to disability.

In an analysis of recent advertising that includes disability images and themes, Beth Haller and Sue Ralph (2006) find that, although more advertising campaigns associate disability with empowerment, pride and inclusion, the tendency to embrace stigmatising and antiquated themes associated with the supercrip and tragedy dominates. A recent advertisement for Guinness leverages the new aesthetic of disabled masculinity; however, it problematically does not conclude by celebrating the achievements of a disabled athlete and instead attempts to reinsert this new discourse into a system of compulsory able-bodiedness (see McRuer, 2006). It begins with a basketball flying towards a hoop but missing the shot. The camera then pans down to show a group of men in wheelchairs aggressively playing basketball, some are high-fiving, others wrestling with each other and the ball, taking shots and missing, falling out of chairs. It is set to opera-style music – *To Build a Home* by The Cinematic Orchestra. Just as the players are getting into the game, one says 'you guys are getting better at this' as the rest stand up and walk off referring to him as 'buddy'. The ad's slogan is 'dedication, loyalty, friendship' and we can infer the men are showing dedication, loyalty and friendship by playing wheelchair basketball with their wheelchair-using friend.

As I have discussed throughout this book, the representation of disability in popular culture has been consistently criticised in the disability studies literature. A key example is example Paul Longmore's 1985 article *Screening Stereotypes* which I introduced in Chapter 4. However, it is important to note that Longmore ended his article with the optimistic suggestion that featuring people with disability in television commercials represented a major departure from more common images of disability which reinforce 'cultural prejudice'. He described a new image of disability he saw emerging through television commercials where people with disabilities are portrayed as 'attractive, active and "with it", involved and competitive' as opposed to 'helpless and dependent'. Similarly, David Hevey (1992), although critical of the continued enfreakment of disability imagery, lamented the lack of disability in commercial advertising.

Although the men in the Guinness advert are attractive, active, involved, competitive and with it, they are predominately able-bodied – the one disabled man is peripheral. As the team go down to the pub for a pint of Guinness the voice over explains that 'the choices we make reveal the true nature of our character'. As such this advert reinforces a system US academic Robert McRuer describes as *compulsory able-bodiedness*. McRuer explains the notion of the 'able body' depend on the ways disability is made visible, including in the Oxford English Dictionary which defines the able body as 'free from disability'. He maintains that this system demands we agree that able-bodiedness is preferable, it becomes 'common sense' that we would all prefer to stand up and walk away from the wheelchairs at the end of the Guinness advert. The men in this advert, shown to be 'free from disability' by standing and walking away, have able bodies. Admittedly, the real wheelchair basketball player is clearly the best player, he blocks the others and never falls out of his chair, yet he cannot make a shot. It is also true that wheelchair basketball teams consisting of both non-disabled and disabled players actually exist, and the one player with an actual disability is definitely 'attractive, active, involved and competitive'; however, the fact that the majority all walk away suggests that able-bodiedness is the foundational identity for athletic men. The advert does, however, draw on discourses of disability and masculinity first introduced in the breakout documentary *Murderball*, a film which aligned disability with hyper masculinity.

You Have to be Disabled to Play this Game: *Murderball*

The 2005 documentary release *Murderball* follows the 2004 US Paralympics wheelchair rugby team as they prepare to face Canada in Athens. The narrative is familiar – a sporting team of intensely masculine men prepare to battle their arch-rivals however, the inclusion and indeed necessity of disability adds a layer of innovation and social critique as the athletes fight against what they see as the discriminatory social beliefs that emasculate them.

This film again illustrates sporting popular culture as an intersection between aesthetics, economics, technology and everyday life. The political conflicts of daily life are played out as heroes and rivals are discursively created and the everyday of disability explored as the elite athletes discuss the ways they are patronised in everyday life through people's low expectations of their ability to navigate the world, drive a car, have sex. A hyper-masculine aesthetic is created through their participation in an aggressive sport. With the wheelchair being the most culturally recognisable technology of disability, the importance of technology to sport is communicated through the highly modified game chairs as the team are variously described as 'gladiators on wheels' and the wheels themselves as Mad Max-style chairs.

Significantly, the documentary also offers the additional information related to aesthetics and emotion which Bertling and Schierl (2008) argue is vital in attracting an audience. Indeed, while not initially commercially successful, *Murderball* was a hit on the festival circuit and made a lasting impact on the cultural zeitgeist as evidenced by the Guinness advert. It won a spate of awards at numerous film festivals, including both the Documentary Audience Award and a Special Jury Prize for Editing at the 2005 Sundance Film Festival. It was also nominated in the documentary category at the Academy Awards in 2006.

The image of a wheelchair in films is an easily recognisable symbol of a performance of disability, a symbol that audience members typically do not desire. However, in *Murderball*, the wheelchair is constructed as an object of desire. Throughout the film, Keith, a recently injured young man offers a parallel story to the murderball team as he adjusts to life with a spinal cord injury. When team captain Mark Zupan visits Keith's rehabilitation hospital, Keith is immediately drawn to Mark's competition chair. His reclaimed masculinity is juxtaposed with the feminising influence of the hospital environment as his nurse and mother attempt to discourage him from riding in the chair. Keith and Zupan laugh at them, asking what's the worst that could happen? Petra Kuppers (2007) describes the wheelchair in this scene as a symbol of 'freedom, sexiness and regained masculinity-maschismo' (p. 81).

This documentary problematises the two most enduring representations of disability – a loss of sexuality and a lack of community – by chronicling the lives of hyper-masculine athletes with disability (Garland-Thomson, 2007). Media images often use disability as an exploration of masculinity and dependency. However, they typically operate in the context of a loss of masculinity. By comparison, *Murderball* repositions the wheelchair away from a loss of masculinity, towards the means of access to a hyper-masculine world – you must be disabled to play murderball. Disability has provided these young men 'a meaningful life in which one thrives rather than languishes' (Garland-Thomson, 2007, p. 115).

Critical Questions

While *Murderball* came at a crucial juncture in disability studies, there are several aspects of this film that warrant further critical investigation. Firstly, disability stigma is neutralised through stereotypes of masculinity, including sexism. At several points throughout the film, women are either ridiculed or sexualised in order to reinforce the dominance of these men. Secondly, the connection between sporting cultures and the myth of control should be interrogated. The focus on sport as a means to regain meaningful social access could reinforce the myth of body control which as discussed has occupied an ominous position over the lives of people with disability.

Finally the film communicated a problematic disregard for the Special Olympics. Although offering an empowering representation of disability in the context of masculinity, the disabled athletes in *Murderball* refused any association with the Special Olympics, a competition established for people with intellectual impairments, and an organisation they see as inferior. To return to Hall's concept of othering, the Special Olympics are constructed as the outsider group, the abnormal to the Murderball 'normal'. Whereas the Paralympic games have long been considered the inferior sporting event in comparison with the Olympics, within the disability sports arena they are considered the best. Indeed the Special Olympics is not given appropriate media coverage (Carter and Williams, 2012).

Conclusion

As I have discussed throughout this book, critical disability studies seek to expose the creation of a normative body. This discipline has both established the way a disabled body is created and, more recently, considered the creation of ableness. By their very nature, all bodies are out of control and people with disability are an acute reminder of the temporariness of an able-bodied ontology. However, although representations of disabled athletes do not typically fit the cultural mythology of strength and super human achievement, the increasing commercialisation of disabled sports provides an opportunity for critical analysis.

Sport is competition, athletes compete against one another to be the best, win the race, take the gold, be number one. By the very definition of sport, certain athletes have the competitive edge, are better than the others. Athletes, like people with disability, deviate from the norm. However, their extraordinary bodies are revered, not subjugated. In many ways sport is about controlling the body, and disabled sports is no different.

Throughout the chapter I discussed Oscar Pistorius as an ambiguous figure in disability sports. While he first came to attention when he sought to compete against able-bodied athletes, the heroic Paralympic narrative built around him is increasingly questioned following his manslaughter conviction.

A number of other athletes, in a number of sports not necessarily of the Paralympic level, have also sought to compete against their able-bodied peers. For example, Deb Roach, a disabled pole dancer, competed against able-bodied competitors in an Australian pole dancing competition in 2009 and won. She describes the importance of pole dancing to her sense of self, 'I have always loved dancing but as a child and teen with low self esteem I believed that aesthetic and athletic pursuits were not for me, not for my "different" body … As an adult, I learned to challenge my assumptions' (Roach cited in Reilly, 2012). Competitors are judged in disabled pole dancing according to different criteria on the basis of their impairment (personal communication). Through an intense exercise regime and routine modification, Roach adapted routines devised by and for two-handed people to suit a one-armed pole dancer such as herself. However, should athletes with disabilities, like Pistorius and Roach, aspire to compete against non-disabled people? Do accommodations or prosthetics put them at an advantage? What does the position of athletes with disability in popular culture tell us about the cultural construction and commodification of disability, or more specifically ability?

Despite this, the classification systems that level the playing field and ensure impairment does not affect the outcome of the competition, characteristic of disability sports, offer an insight into the potential to redesign environments to allow for the participation of people with disability. However, sport, especially commercial sport, is not spontaneous – a number of social roles and rituals pervade sport as popular culture. While disability sports is increasingly gaining an audience through the embrace of aesthetics in campaigns like *Meet the Superhumans* and the documentary film *Murderball*, the supercrip image continues to articulate a clearly defined role for people with disability.

Disability sports both reveal and maintain the production of ableism. Sport's broader focus on controlling the body and the creation of the normate is an example of the cultural and institutional reinforcement of ableism. Yet, the classification system and prosthetics that allow disabled athletes to compete in sport in such a way that their impairment does not affect the 'outcome' demonstrates that society can be redesigned to allow a fuller inclusion of people with bodies that deviate from 'the norm'.

Chapter 8
Disability and Spreadable Media: Access, Representation and Inspiration Porn

On 1 October 2009, Courtney, a writer at the influential Feminist blog site *Feministing*, posted a story about chivalry that included the statement, '… if having my car door opened makes me feel like lover man thinks I'm an invalid, not so feminist' (Courtney, 2009a). The blog was a short but stimulating piece about gender roles, within heterosexual romantic love designed to elicit discussion about whether equality can coexist with chivalry. However, Courtney's casual use of the word invalid angered a number of *Feministing* readers who identified as feminists with disabilities.

Initially responding as individuals, several commented on Courtney's post, others sent emails to the *Feministing* editors, some did both. Then blogger s.e. smith decided to make the complaint public and wrote an 'open letter' encouraging others to repost it on their sites as co-signers. smith's open letter summarised the disabled feminists' ongoing issues with *Feministing*:

> You have a pretty poor track record on even covering disability issues, and the casual ableism which I see in your comment threads and sometimes in your very posts is extremely grating. It is especially irritating to see dismissive responses from site administrators when this issue is brought up … Please address this. Feminism includes people with disabilities. Disability is a feminist issue. Please make Feministing more inclusionary. (s.e. smith, 2009)

As Courtney and smith communicated via email over what to do next – start a discussion thread, create a roundtable discussion or schedule a chat between *Feministing* writers and the disabled feminists – smith's open letter spread rapidly across the blogosphere and the disabled feminists mobilised. Another blogger reposted the open letter to the *Feministing* site itself where discussions became, in the words of *Feministing* creator Jessica Valenti, 'extremely hostile' (Valenti cited in s.e. smith, 2009). Valenti closed the discussion and smith encouraged patience as the group of feminists with disability entered discussions with *Feministing* writers and editors about how to address ableism within the feminist blogosphere.

The future looked promising as a chat was set up; however, following discussions, disquiet continued on a number of sites and discussion forums, with the much anticipated chat variously described as a joke, lip-service, condescending and rude. By comparison, Courtney updated the *Feministing* community with her version of events:

> We moved forward by scheduling an online chat between these activists, who meanwhile started their own blog (their abelist [sic] word profiles are really enlightening, as are their regular recommended readings, and fantastic general content), [and Feministing staff]. It was a productive and affirming experience for me personally. This group of activists and bloggers communicated their suggestions with incredible clarity and coordination, and as it turns out, most of their ideas were things that [writers at Feministing] were either already discussing or open to implementing. (Courtney, 2009b)

However, Courtney went on to describe the exchange as 'empowering' and used other language that the group of disability bloggers felt was inappropriate and again illustrative of casual ableism. The disabled feminists joined together to form a new blog – *Feminists with Disability for a Way Forward (FWD)* – to shape and promote the disability movement online and encourage disability voices in debates from which disability is usually silenced. The site ran from 2009 to 2011.

Consider the story from Courtney's point of view. She was writing for possibly the most important feminist publication of recent years and used what she must have considered a neutral word to describe a feeling of powerlessness. But the word invalid is not neutral. In the context of disability, a complex cultural history exists and Courtney's casual use of the word is an example of Mitchell and Snyder's (2000) observation that disability is often constructed by other marginalised groups, including feminists, as 'the real limitation from which they must escape' (p. 2). The word invalid, derived from the Latin *invalidus* meaning 'not strong, infirm, weak, inadequate' was initially used as an adjective during the 1600s. However, within a short period of time, the word was in use as a noun to describe people 'infirm from sickness or disease; enfeebled or disabled by illness or injury' (Dictionary). Given that the disability pension was at one point called the invalid pension and an entry in the Oxford English Dictionary describes the transport of disabled soldiers as the transports of invalids suggests people with disability have historically been considered as being without value (Dictionary). As I discussed in Chapter 4, the 1997 film *Gattaca* ironically uses this word to describe people who would be considered non-disabled now to critique the increasing post-human approach to conception and work.

The intense medicalisation of disability along with disability's cultural devaluation, even by those groups undertaking a similar cultural fight for equality, explain Courtney's description of the exchange as empowering and personally satisfying. However, the feminists with disability did not appreciate the condescending tone when they sought only to reveal disability as a feminist issue. Discussions of the exchange can be found on smith's blog site at http://meloukhia.net/2009/10/an_open_letter_to_feministing/and from the point of view of *Feministing* at http://feministing.com/2009/10/28/follow-up-on-disability-rights-dialogue/comment-page-1/. Other links such as the chat transcript and the 'hostile' discussion have gone cold. These archives attest to the rapid spread of online media and activism, with *FWD* appearing less than a month after *Feministing*'s initial offensive post.

The emergence of *FWD* through tensions within the feminist blogosphere is a story about many things – Courtney's lack of understanding of disability issues, reflexive ableism even within feminist discussion, smith's influence as a blogger, a mobilisation of disability rights – but one of the most significant themes running through the story is the power of collective intelligence in the spread of media online.

Collective intelligence is a form of collaboration where people with both more and less experience with a topic such as disability come together in online spaces, as in the case of the *Feministing/FWD* tension, to assist one another in making sense of the issue. According to French cyber theorist Pierre Lévy (1997), even those views that may be deemed ignorant or 'other' offer an opportunity to gain new knowledge and test ideas. Courtney's use of the word invalid to describe female disempowerment provided the opportunity for an entire online community to gain new knowledge about ableism as well as another niche community to gain traction and spread influence. As a site of cultural mediation these discussions reflect current attitudes regarding disability.

Although smith describes failing to change the culture of ableism at *Feministing*, the bloggers were able to set up their own site, which became an influential publication in its own right. Thus, as a disability blogosphere cohered through debate and tension within the feminist blogosphere, *FWD* became what Yochachi Benkler (2006) describes as a superstar blog. Blogs maintain cultural influence through communities of interest which become highly connected through hyperlinks. Benkler describes blogs on the same topics as clusters. Clusters connect as communities by engaging in collective intelligence to filter relevant views. These clusters become highly specific in their views as groups of people with common interests to join together under 'superstar' blogs, offering a strategy of media distribution and exchange. Superstar blogs articulate dominant views and create 'shortcuts to wide attention' (p. 13). Under Benkler's framework, the feminist blogosphere would be described as a cluster and *Feministing* as a superstar blog. Superstar blogs are especially important when clusters service increasingly small or niche communities of interest such as *FWD* did.

With popular culture increasingly taking on a new media infrastructure, new media theories such as collective intelligence and spreadable media become significant to a discussion of disability. This chapter explores disability's central role in what Henry Jenkins, Sam Ford and Joshua Green describe as 'spreadable media', a phenomenon that is changing the makeup of the media industry. Spreadable media is the forwarding and sharing of news stories or videos among a person's network via social networking and email (see Jenkins, 2013). Jenkins et al. draw on John Fiske's definition of popular culture as producerly to argue that spreadable media *is* popular culture. Whereas messages are encoded into media content, audiences derive meaning from them and use popular culture in their own lives for their own purposes. Although Courtney was attempting to elicit a discussion of chivalry as potentially (dis)empowering for women, the disabled feminists interpreted the her use of the word invalid as a continuation of the cultural dislocation felt by people with disability. The discussion was considered sufficiently important to spread throughout the blogosphere and result in the creation of a new superstar blog to discuss these and other cultural issues from a disability perspective. Media that spreads is open to interpretation and allows audiences to 'pluralize the meanings and pleasures [mass culture] offers, evade or resist its disciplinary efforts, fracture its homogeneity or coherence, raid or poach upon its terrain' (Fiske, 1989 cited in Jenkins, 2013, p. 200). Producerly content is incorporated into people's lives in ways that are meaningful to them. This fracturing and then rejoining of the feminist and disabled feminist blogospheres also highlights the significance of niche audiences in a new media environment.

Throughout this chapter I consider what happens to producerly popular culture when it encounters new media digitisation. While there is much opportunity for a social and cultural interrogation of disability, there also remain problematic contradictions, schisms, and new modes of exploitation that disempower both the disabled and non-disabled. The chapter begins by discussing the potential for collective intelligence in the use of new media as participatory culture. Drawing on Bruns' concept of produsage, I locate this tendency as a precursor to spreadable media. This section considers the disability blogosphere and disability blog carnivals in particular as they contribute to both the spread of new ways of understanding disability and to disability readings of popular culture. The section concludes with a discussion of charity and pity as two entrenched cultural discourses that continue to be applied to and shape the disability experience.

The chapter then moves to consider the increasing importance of spreadable media in the current online environment. Whereas charity discourses are often criticised for their impacts on disability, and how the experience of disability is understood, this section reveals the way these long-standing images of disability are being leveraged through spreadable media as users become a commodity bought and sold on an underground marketplace. The section interrogates in particular the way 'inspirational' images of disability and terminal illnesses are used on the social networking site Facebook to 'farm likes'.

The chapter continues the discussion of inspirational images of disability to bring together participatory cultures and spreadable media to offer a case study analysis of the rise and critique of so-called 'inspiration porn'. There is a robust discussion taking place on blogs and social media regarding the inspirational framing of people with disability. While new media has certainly increased the opportunity for inspirational images of disability to be viewed by large and varied populations, it has also allowed the spread of views that critique and interrogate this seemingly natural paradigm of disability.

The chapter then discusses people with disability making and distributing web series online as an example of an alternative media world, outside the confines of media framing, ritual and hierarchy. Despite the opportunity for greater inclusion, a number of inherent contradictions and ambiguities continue to surround this claim. New media is often celebrated for including everyone and for making popular culture accessible. The chapter concludes with reflections regarding accessibility and the reproduction of disabling practices, attitudes and organisations online.

Participatory Culture: Here Comes Everybody

The notion that 'everybody' can participate online pervades enthusiastic discussions of new media, particularly following web 2.0 which can be broadly defined as online practices which rely and thrive on the collaboration and participation of its users. This discourse dominates academic and industry discussions alike. For example, Clay Shirky titled his book, which looks at the power of online group action, *Here Comes Everybody*, and Mark Zuckerberg describes his motivations for creating Facebook as wanting people to better connect to the world around them and often espouses the importance of network connection, for everybody. With cyberspace becoming less the stuff of science fiction and more and more ubiquitous in our lives, it is also becoming easier to use. As Denise Stokes explains in an article about people with disabilities' use of Facebook and blog sites, 'it really is as simple as that. A ten-year-old will tell you a four-year-old can do it' (Stokes, 2008, p. 16).

Claims of accessibility and the propensity for everybody to be involved also pervades the 'about' sections of the most popular social networking sites. The microblogging site Twitter claims to enable the sharing of information without barriers, while YouTube 'allows billions of people to discover, watch and share originally-created videos' (YouTube, 2014). Wikipedia celebrates the fact that anyone with an internet connection can create or make changes to an entry, and

Tumblr claims to empower ordinary people. As Jenkins et al. (2013) observe, users, consumers and audiences have been repositioned as co-creators who 'upload, tag, organize, and categorize content on YouTube, Flickr, and a myriad of other sites' (p. 49).

Henry Jenkins (2006) draws on the work of Pierre Lévy to argue that people with disparate beliefs and experiences engage in collective meaning making to leverage (their) combined expertise and offer both new texts and new ways of understanding existing texts (p. 17). The ubiquity of the web in our lives is described as creating a never before seen social inclusion, where it would seem anyone can participate in the production and consumption of media and popular culture. However, this concept of accessibility and the opportunity for everyone to get involved and contribute is problematic when it comes to the inclusion of people with disability, a concept I discuss later in the chapter.

In *Collective Intelligence, Mankind's Emerging World in Cyberspace*, Pierre Lévy argues that the computerisation of society will 'promote the construction of intelligent communities in which our social and cognitive potential can be mutually developed and enhanced' (Lévy, 1997, p. 17). When more people become connected and participate in sharing knowledge within and across networks, more comprehensive information on particular issues will emerge. As Lévy explains, 'no one knows everything, everyone knows something' (p. 13). Indeed, with *Feministing* attempting to reveal the ways women are disempowered through routine cultural practices, the disabled feminists were able to offer a more comprehensive view of this picture through their argument that ableist language is a continuation of the cultural disempowerment imposed upon women. Learning from each other is central to Lévy's information utopia and holds significant potential to disability as popular culture increasingly takes on a new media infrastructure.

Lévy emphasises the need for collaborative efforts and collective intelligence in the exchange of information and knowledge (p. 13). He maintains that much can be learnt and gained even from people judged 'ignorant' (p. 14) through a collaborative approach to knowledge acquisition. The result could bring about the next phase of intellectual and social evolution. With the rise of online newspapers, television companion websites, Facebook fan pages, popular culture blogs and trending topics on Twitter, Lévy's insights hold particular significance as active audiences, publics and users become creative in their engagement in a process of collective intelligence.

This online content is created by people journalist Dan Gillmore describes as 'the former audience' (cited in Shirky, 2008, p. 7). Whereas the audience used to wait for the media, or popular culture to come to them, the former audience now participates in its creation. While much online conversation appears casual, gossipy and perhaps even the trashiest of popular culture, drawing on Fiske's conception of gossip culture as producerly, we can see that even a bemused engagement with disability popular culture online stimulates new meanings. Produsers (or producer-users) and wreaders (writer-readers) are two terms often applied to the former audience's online engagement. The interaction is much more active than previous modes of media and, in the case of blogging for example, wrestles the mode of production away from media heavyweights towards a more participatory context.

Disability Blogosphere

The blogosphere has been attributed with democratising the media industry, of providing people with non-mainstream or peripheral views and identities an opportunity for publication. Blog carnivals are community-based projects where a blogger solicits other blogs around a similar theme and then publishes a link to selected blogs under the same topic on their own blog. Blog carnivals offer another opportunity for interconnection between individual blogs within communities through hyperlinks, and help establish the importance of particular blogs and particular issues within blog clusters.

A disability blog carnival centrally organised by the School of Disability Studies at Temple University in Philadelphia was first launched in 2006 and ran until 2012 when it closed in recognition that the online environment had shifted from blogs towards other formats such as social networking (Richards, 2012). However, the 84 carnivals which did run provide, in the words of curator Penny Richards, 'a strong record of disability blogosphere for a vibrant six years'. They also provide a diverse insight to the different ways people with disabilities use the blogging format to engage with the media to open up new paradigms of understanding disability in media and culture. Despite the proliferation of other online venues and formats, which I will discuss later in this chapter, as Scott Hollier (2012) explains in his review of people with disabilities' use of social networking, blogging remains 'a useful ... way to reflect on disability-related issues' (p. 31).

Further, 6 years' worth of disability blog carnivals provide an important insight into the ways blogs provide accessible explanations of complex disability theories through an embrace of both personal experience and an interrogation of the effects of a disabling world. Thoreau describes this as a 'personal narrative' model of disability, and sees it running through the disability blogosphere (Thoreau, 2006). An engagement with popular culture, both disability- and non-disability-themed, offer important insights into the experience of disability. For example, the January 2011 blog carnival theme borrowed from the Shrek theme song *Let Your Freak Flag Fly*. Bloggers were asked to submit blogs related to proudly identifying as a person with disability:

Write about a time when you openly and proudly identified as a person with a disability, or, if you're a non-disabled ally, write about a time when you were proud to stand by us. Or ….you could make it into a musing on the word "freak" itself, and related words. Do they help us? Hurt us? Is it wrong to call ourselves freaks, spazzes, and gimps? Or is it empowering? Or … something else!! (Liebowitz, 2010a)

The personal narrative model of disability can be seen in these blog carnivals as the entries introduce readers to political aspects of disability and identity. For example, entries in the November 2010 carnival 'Intersections' take a political stance to disability – and are embedded in cultural studies:

The point is disability is an interesting enough societal issue as it is, when it's combined with other "strikes", so to speak, it becomes even more interesting. Intersection theory, as we learned in sociology, explores the meeting point between social class, gender, race, etc. Of course disability was nowhere mentioned, but then again, that's our job as disability bloggers, to bring disability out of the woodwork. We're highlighting disability as a unique sociological issue, an issue as important as social class, gender, and race. We are shedding light on one of the experiences most feared by society – and providing insight into a striking new world. (Liebowitz, 2010b)

This is an accessible explanation of the critical study of disability and introduces a narrative about disability that is rarely acknowledged. Personal perspectives, welcomed within the blogosphere, are important especially when they intersect with other cultural theories:

Disability has emotional baggage and to help me because I am disabled is an act of nobility, compassion and generosity. [Some people] may be no more capable of, say, setting up an e-mail account than I am capable of driving or using public transport to get to where I want to go, but because I am disabled, their giving me a lift becomes an act of heroism my amateur techy skills can't compete with. Such attitudes are a real problem, because quite apart from having to deal with someone who treats you like they're carrying you on their back up a mountain, they invest you and your impairments with so much emotional baggage. With tragedy, helplessness and dependence which is not your own. (The Goldfish, 2010)

The Goldfish distils complex academic theories around stigma using real world examples in this blog entry. Everyone, including both people with disability and those without, are dependent to a certain extent. This 'interdependence' can relate to technology, skills, abilities and disabilities. However, as The Goldfish finds, cultural discourses of disability see (him) being treated as less than or more dependent than a non-disabled person who may behave in a similar way in a different context. The Goldfish's example of discriminatory social attitudes is illuminating – while a person with disability is pitied or interpreted as tragic for not being able to drive, a non-disabled person who cannot fix a computer is not considered helpless in the same way. That is to say, the extent to which a person is disabled relies on expectations that already exist in society. To conclude, these personal narrative blogs, linking disability activism and experience through carnivals, reveal disability as a complex identity constituted by both physical difference and social stigma.

Spreadable Media

Henry Jenkins, Sam Ford and Joshua Green (2013) argue that we are witnessing a more participatory (and messy) era of culture through 'spreadable media' (p. 2). Spreadable media is the forwarding and sharing of news stories or videos among a person's network via social networking and email (see Jenkins, 2013). Media is unbound to geographical locations, and the popularity of popular culture becomes dependent on the endorsement of people within a network. Disability features heavily in spreadable media, often due to its emotive influence. This is not unique to new media content, however; disability has long been used in popular culture to evoke emotion by leveraging 'longstanding associations of stigma with bodily difference' (Snyder and Mitchell, 2010, p. 192). In the context of photographic news media, Beth Haller (2000) has previously observed that if 'they limp, they lead', meaning disability takes prime place in news coverage in order to attract an audience (Haller, 2000).

An image, video or link that has spread rapidly through numerous internet populations through social networking and email is often described as going 'viral'. Some examples of disability in spreadable media that have gone viral include Susan Boyle's audition for *Britain's Got Talent*, a YouTube video of a young boy with cerebral palsy competing at his school athletics carnival, a Canadian mother's response to a neighbour's note demanding she keep her autistic daughter out of public view, 'Mallory' the girl with Down's Syndrome whose brother requested Facebook likes to prove she was beautiful, and, as I write this chapter, footage of two teenaged girls assaulting an elderly man with vision impairment on public transport.

These are but a few examples of disability in spreadable media, a new phenomenon in cultural production and exchange that is refiguring the way we think about popular culture. Individuals make decisions about spreading

147

this media among their networks. Some content begins as amateur, user-generated content, while others are uploaded (or leveraged) by professional news organisations. More still, such as the Mallory example (which I will discuss later in the chapter), are a hoax designed to attract Facebook likes for insidious money-making purposes.

Spreadable media illustrates the way our emotions are leveraged in popular culture. We spread media because it either makes us think or makes us feel … or makes us think by making us feel. Jenkins et al. (2013) locate Susan Boyle's audition video as a particularly significant moment in the shift towards spreadable media. David Calvert (2013) similarly highlights the importance of Boyle's audition on *Britain's Got Talent* to discerning a televisual shift in the representation of disability. Boyle initially auditioned for a geographically-restricted television program – only people in the UK could watch *Britain's Got Talent*. However, following her audition performance of *I Dreamed a Dream*, the so-called former audience began uploading videos of it to the internet and sharing it among their networks on sites such as Facebook and Twitter. Within 9 days Boyle had become an international sensation, with over 100 million viewers watching her audition video (Dobuzinskis, 2009). Through spreadable media Boyle has been able to maintain her significance long past the 15 minutes of fame usually afforded to those who compete in reality television singing contests. Although people spreading her video were not initially aware of her disability, they were aware of her outsider status and Boyle did not lose popularity when her disability was revealed.

Perhaps disability had nothing to do with people's motivations for spreading Boyle's *I Dreamed a Dream*; however, when it was revealed, the performance took on a new meaning. The shift of messages encoded *into* mass culture towards meanings taken *from* popular culture took on a new form for people, who began discussing what Boyle's disability meant to how they viewed their own lives:

> The more I play her video and listen to her singing, the more I grow to admire this most unassuming lady. Susan is the model and heroine of the normal masses … the majority of us who have ordinary lives, doing ordinary things and may be old, disabled, unemployed, fat, etc. … She brings hope and light. What a lady! (ngayonatkailanman, 2009, 13 April)

Following recent news articles revealing Boyle's diagnosis of Asperger's syndrome, people engaged in conversations about news framing of disability, the removal of Asperger's from the Diagnostic and Statistical Manual of Mental Disorders in favour of an autism severity ranking, and whether a diagnosis was useful or more damaging to the way disability is experienced (see Deveney, 2013). These commenters were using the spread of popular culture – from a geographically-restricted television show, to international superstardom, to an online newspaper – to discuss issues relevant to the social positioning of disability. In other words, they were engaging in a process of collective intelligence.

Inspiration Porn

In 2013, when the Australian Prime Minister at the time, Kevin Rudd, patted a woman with a disability on the head while giving her a cuddle, a robust debate erupted on Twitter among key figures of the Australian disability community, feminists and political reporters. The photo opportunity came after Rudd launched Australia's first disability insurance scheme.

Disability advocate Stella Young took to Twitter to describe the photo opportunity as leaving her 'shaking with rage', while comedian Joe Hildebrand ridiculed her on Twitter and accused her of never being happy. He followed the Twitter disagreement up with an opinion piece in *The Telegraph* where he asked 'what precisely the point of her outrage' was:

> It is fair to ask that if a smiling Prime Minister and a laughing woman embracing each other to celebrate the introduction of the National Disability Insurance Scheme leaves Stella "shaking with rage", what exactly does it take to make her happy? (Hildebrand, 2013)

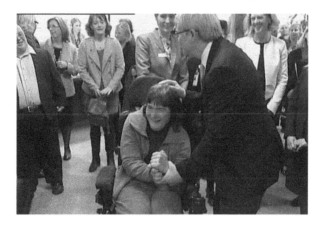

Figure 8.1   Prime Minister Kevin Rudd pats a woman on the head at the launch of DisabilityCare Australia 11 July 2013

Source: © ABC Australia.

He went on to accuse her of being an extremist on the hunt for something to be upset about:

> One unfortunate conclusion is that she never will be. Rather that she, like many on the extreme left, and indeed the extreme right – neither of which are any friends of mine – will never be happy. Instead both sets of malcontents seem to prefer to pore through any trough of information searching for things to be upset about. (Hildebrand, 2013)

Those of us in disability studies would describe Hildebrand as ignorant when it comes to disability. However, drawing on Lévy's (1997) argument, Hildebrand's views offer an important moment for collective intelligence. His attack on Young drew attention to the way the 'disability as inspirational' paradigm has been naturalised as common sense and entrenched in our culture. The online debate also reveals a key shift between older and newer media forms, with traditional news framing techniques such as the happy prime minister embracing the poor person with disability for whom we should feel only pity and charity, towards people with disability articulating the problem with this image, towards others heavily invested in maintaining the cultural dislocation of disability as inspirational tragedy.

Intriguingly, Young had published a piece about this very issue only the year before. She could have been describing her (future) exchange with Hildebrand when she argued:

> Most journalists seem utterly incapable of writing or talking about a person with a disability without using phrases like "overcoming disability", "brave", "suffers from", "defying the odds", "wheelchair bound" or, my personal favourite, "inspirational".
> If we even begin to question the way we're labelled, we slide immediately to the other end of the scale and become "bitter" and "ungrateful". We fail to be what people expect. (Young, 2012)

Young was describing a phenomenon she calls *inspiration porn* where images of people with disability are constructed as inspirational in order to make the non-disabled feel better about themselves:

> Inspiration porn is an image of a person with a disability, often a kid, doing something completely ordinary – like playing, or talking, or running, or drawing a picture, or hitting a tennis ball – carrying a caption like "your excuse is invalid" or "before you quit, try". Let me be clear about the intent of this inspiration porn; it's there so that non-disabled people can put their worries into perspective. So they can go, "Oh well if that kid who doesn't have any legs can smile while

he's having an awesome time, I should never, EVER feel bad about my life". It's there so that non-disabled people can look at us and think "well, it could be worse … I could be that person".

To draw on Jenkins' (2006) spreadable media framework, Young's piece was 'sticky' – it spread quickly and significantly went viral, and the term 'inspiration porn' entered the popular critical disability zeitgeist. Immediately following its initial publication on the disability-specific site *Ramp Up*, Young's article was republished on a number of other sites and initiated an enduring discussion on both disability and mainstream blogs about the problematic ways disability is represented in the media and viewed in society. Arguments for and against the inspirational discourse surrounding disability were offered, and the conversation continues on a number of personal blogging sites.

Quentin Kenihan, who appeared on the Australian program *A Current Affair* throughout the 1980s in 'inspirational' stories, weighed into the debate at *Ramp Up*:

I see nothing wrong with Disabled people inspiring others. I don't see anything wrong with anyone finding inspiration in something or someone as long as it makes that person want to do better in life. No one should ever be hounded, bullied or shunned for being inspired nor finding inspiration in something or someone. (Quentin comment on Young, 2012)

Kenihan described Young's argument as 'silly'. However, Young's original publication generated 199 comments on *Ramp Up*, it then elicited 93 when it was republished on *The Drum* and 157 on *Mamamia*. While these numbers may be considered low in the overall context of spreadable media, they reveal the importance of media spreading among niche groups, or clusters. The term 'inspiration porn' has therefore had longevity and continues to be actively debated within the disability blogosphere and referred back to on feminist sites such as *Destroy The Joint* and even within the Television Without Pity (TWOP) discussion of *Push Girls* analysed in Chapter 5.

Other commenters to a similar blog published by Phillipa Willits on *The Independent* the subsequent month drew attention to the 'negative' nature of the argument and problematic use of the word porn. They illustrate Jenkins' conception of collective intelligence to show that people experience disability, and the cultural messages that surround it, in different ways:

I personally think this article is a gross overreaction to an image that was simply made to make people feel good. As someone with only minor disabilities, I can see how, if taken the wrong way, this image could be upsetting, but honestly why over-think it that much? The quotation is simply delivering a positive

151

message, to even those who are disabled, not to consider their disability when trying their very hardest. A man without legs could just as easily become an extremely successful lawyer as he could an Olympian, and it's silly to assume that it only refers to physical accomplishments. I think the picture is trying to say that no matter what you can't do, there's always something that you can do. Whether it be painting, writing, speaking, running, or even something as simple as playing a video game, there is always something you can succeed at as long as you have a "good attitude". I just think that this article is much too negative. (James Abbaticchio comment on Willitts, 2012)

Both Young and Willitts made explicit reference to Oscar Pistorius photos doing the rounds on Facebook in their articles. Other commenters accused Willitts of 'overthinking' the issue of disability and of displaying a negative attitude. Yet people are culturally wedded to the concept that people with disability are inspirational. Although the inspirational photos of Pistorius that Young and Willitts criticise have lost cultural significance and become almost non-existent since his arrest and subsequent conviction, 'cripspiration' (Willitts) and inspiration porn (Young) continues to pervade spreadable media. These images have taken on an even more sinister significance than simply making the non-disabled feel better about themselves – they are being used as click bait in the commodification of sympathy.

Liking to be Liked

As Facebook solidifies its dominance in our methods of communication, people are devising insidious ways to make money in this arena. Whereas users think about Facebook in terms of the *social* and the ephemeral nature of communication in particular, Facebook and other business focus on the *media* aspect (Leaver, 2013b) and where money can be made. Facebook may be free to use; however, users are in effect bought and sold for the personal information they share. This information is big business.

Existential guilt appeal, or the comparison of one's own well-being to those of others, is a successful tool employed by charities to elicit donations (Lwin and Phau, 2008). Jennifer Aaker and Andy Smith (2010), authors of *The Dragonfly Effect*, encourage businesses engaging in new media platforms to create a sense of community by cultivating a sense of social good. They note that when people to give to charity the areas of their brain associated with selfish pleasures are activated. This activation of pleasure and the experience of existential guilt is also being leveraged by insidious marketers and scammers on Facebook, with taglines accompanying spreadable images of disability such as:

Like if you hate cancer, ignore if you don't

This is my sister Mallory. She has Down syndrome and doesn't think she's beautiful. Please like this photo so I can show her later that she truly is beautiful Like if You Respect him, ignore if you don't

These pages are created for the purposes of a new phenomenon called 'like farming'. This marketing strategy begins when someone creates a page and posts 'innocent' content such as inspirational images. If a Facebook user 'likes' the page, it begins appearing in their newsfeed and also the newsfeeds of their network of friends. The more likes and comments a page gets, the more powerful it becomes in the Facebook 'like algorithm'. The images used by these pages are selected for the visual and emotional cues they offer in the same way that news images of people with disability are selected. Technology blogger Laura Phillips describes the ways these pages have infiltrated her newsfeed:

Every day my (occasionally) informative Facebook news feed is sprinkled with a generous pinch of puppies (sometimes poorly or disabled), strangers' babies (sometimes poorly or disabled), and soldiers (nearly always poorly or disabled) … do you see a theme running here? All of these images were designed to pull at the heart strings and emotionally coerce you into liking the picture presented, some even going so far as to label, insult or even threaten you if you do not comply. (Phillips, 2012)

The more likes/shares/comments a page gets, the more exposure it is given within a particular network. The Facebook like algorithm decides if content is of value to its users. Each page is given an edge rank or score which dictates how much exposure a page is given in other people's newsfeeds. Popularity increases through likes, which also increase the monetary value of a page. Although selling on a page contravenes Facebook's terms of service, a thriving underground market exists where prices are calculated on a '$ per K' basis.

Although these scams are well documented in trade and news publications, they continue to exist on Facebook feeds. Take Mallory for example. The image is of a cute young girl with Down's syndrome wearing glasses and a pink tracksuit. The suggestion that she does not consider herself beautiful leverages all those same emotions that encourage people to contribute to charity. Pages are typically sold on when they reach 100,000 likes (Pearce, 2012). Mallory attracted almost 4 million likes before Terri Johnson, the little girl's real mother, exposed the hoax:

I began receiving strange emails that my daughter "Mallory" had her picture posted on facebook and the picture had gone viral. I thought it was a misunderstanding because I don't have a daughter by that name. Eventually, I was sent a link to a post where I saw a picture of our daughter Katie in a bizarre and crazy technological phenomenon that rocked our simple little world. Katie's picture had been stolen, her identity falsified and a story contrived all for the thrill, challenge and intent of creating a viral post. The reality that someone would exploit our daughter and her special needs for facebook "likes" was nonsensical and surreal. (Johnson, 2012)

While Katie's picture was eventually taken down, more than 6 months after Johnson first alerted Facebook to the issue, another image, one of Merlin German – a wounded soldier with burns over 97 per cent of his body who died in 2008 – continues to circulate. Examples like these make like farming the 'social spam' of spreadable media. Fake charities and other bogus Facebook pages use images of disability and statements about terminal illness to trick people into spreading media content.

The (Alternative) Media World and the Disability Social Agenda

Significantly, however, people with disability are creating and contributing their own media and popular culture to tell new stories and old stories in a new way, outside of the confines of the media world. This media contests the view that disability is a tragedy or an inspiration and that there are either deserving or undeserving people with disability.

In his 2002 book *The Place of Media Power: Pilgrims and Witnesses of the Media Age*, media and communications scholar Nick Couldry explores what happens when 'ordinary people' interact with the media. His book draws on a distinction between the ordinary world and the media world. He argues that the media can shape and maintain what you believe by constructing social reality and setting an agenda. For Couldry, we live our mundane everyday lives in the 'ordinary world', while the media world possesses vast technical and symbolic resources which are leveraged to dictate our interpretations of social life. The media world is exciting and powerful, it's larger than life – ordinary people do not exist in the media world. As I discussed in Chapter 3, the media derives its power to influence the way we think about a number of people, events and social realities through media framing, ritual and hierarchy (Couldry and Curran, 2003). People with disability are therefore turning to internet platform enabled webseries to tell new types of stories about disability, that is outside the confines, framing and hierarchy of the media world.

As people with disability engage in both the productive and consumptive activities of online media, they help shape a shared understanding of disability issues. Nick Couldry and James Curran describe these new opportunities as an *alternative media world*, not imbued with the same powers as the media world but still able to challenge the concentration of media power (Couldry and Curran, 2003). Webseries for example are 'linear digital media created specifically for web distribution' (Leaver, 2013a, p. 161). Disability features in several webseries such as *The Specials* and *My Gimpy Life*. These series – which possess high production values and are distributed online – are discussed below.

Webseries

The Specials – a web series about five young adults with intellectual disabilities who live in a share house in Brighton, UK – began as an example of this new style of media. 'Housemates' Sam, Hilly, Lewis, Megan and Lucy have been friends since childhood and throughout the series experience 'good times and bad times' (episode 1). The series follows a reality TV format with the friends being referred to as 'housemates' and recognisable scenes such as Sam confronting ex-girlfriend Lucy in his underwear (episode 1), Lucy being concerned that her black bra shows through her white t-shirt (episode 2), romantic rejection (episodes 1, 4 and 6), awkward first dates (episode 3), boy problems (episode 3) and housemate love triangles (episodes 9 and 10). *The Specials* has been positively reviewed for offering a non-medicalised representation of people with disability engaging in ordinary behaviours (Shaw, 2010).

My *Gimpy Life* takes a more overt stance towards disability oppression through its humorous critique of disabling attitudes and inaccessible environments. The series follows Teal Sherer, an aspiring actress who uses a wheelchair as she attempts to break into Hollywood. She encounters obstacles everywhere, from not being able to enter inaccessible buildings where both her manager and auditions are located (episode 1), to a lack of disability-specific jobs (episode 2 and 3), to being booked in a 'movement class' to using a toilet as a dressing room and being exploited at work. Episode 3 offers a sophisticated critique of the disability as inspirational paradigm. When Teal completes a poor audition for what appears to be a Black feminist theatre company, the director invites Teal to see the closing night of her latest play *For Colored Girls*. Throughout the evening a number of actors and patrons condescend Teal, describe her as inspirational and tell her they are praying for her. Teal eventually confronts the groups with their prejudice by making a parallel with historical well-meaning racial discrimination:

> That's it, I'm out of here. It's enough! I'm an actress; I didn't come here to be your mascot. Oh you're so so inspiring, such an inspiration. Do you know how insulting that is? It's like me telling her that you're so well spoken or that you could pass for white or that this is just a wonderful little feminist fubu theatre company. (Episode 3 'Inspirational')

Her social life also offers a biting commentary on disability inclusion as she is asked in the street if she can have sex, attends a blind date in an accessible restaurant that turns out to be inaccessible, and inadvertently enters into a relationship with a 'devotee' who actually wants a ménage-à-trois with her wheelchair. According to Jeffrey Hart (2009), digital content for 'niche' audiences tends to be 'edgier' than video designed for consumption via mass audiences (p. 131). *My Gimpy Life* and *The Specials* seek out these niche audiences and make 'edgy' comments on social disablement, living with an impairment, and trying to do ordinary things. Felicia Day's *The Guild* also features disabled actress Teal Sherer in a role.

My Gimpy Life is distributed on YouTube, a video platform often described as accessible by new media theorists and academics working in disability communications alike. However, as a visual medium, YouTube is inaccessible to people with vision impairments.

Disabling New Media

Before concluding this chapter, there are two points about disability in new media that I wish to briefly consider and problematise – accessibility and the opportunity to identify as non-disabled online. While the news media typically celebrates the potential digital technologies holds for the social inclusion of people with disability, theorists within critical disability and internet studies recognise that much of what disables people with disability in the analogue world is carried across to the digital. Attitudes, stereotypes and the absence of core infrastructure are once again a major problem as Ellis and Kent explain:

> Once a piece of information or content is digitised its form is significantly transformed. Whereas a work written on a page is locked in that format, once a word is a digital file it can be transformed to suit any person trying to access it. It can appear as the written word, it can be automatically translated into another language, it can be interpreted as an image, it can be shown in sign language and it can displayed on a Braille tablet. Once that file is connected to the internet all these different modes of access can take place simultaneously, all over the world. This information can be requested through a traditional keyboard, by speech, through eye tracking software or by moving any of a number of different mouse devices. Making that content accessible is a choice. Making it inaccessible is also a choice. (Ellis and Kent, 2011, p. 148)

Ellis and Kent argue that, despite an opportunity to foster a greater inclusion of people with disability – through an increased access to alternative formatting for example – accessibility standards are not observed and, as web 2.0 becomes increasingly graphic dense, people with disability are again excluded through a lack of commitment to social inclusion.

Online environments which allow people with disability to manifest as though non-disabled are also celebrated for the social inclusion they offer for people with disability who are frequently marginalised for how they look. Unlike actual physical (or face-to-face) encounters where physical cues related to disability are, most of the time, obvious, the anonymity of the web allows people to manifest as they please.

However, this is not an empowering long term strategy. I return again to the feminist blogosphere with which I began this chapter. Feminist blogger, columnist and author Laurie Penny questions the rhetoric that the internet is for 'everyone'. She argues that the internet 'was for boys, and if you weren't one you had to pretend to be' (Penny, 2013, p. 4). Clay Shirky (2008) describes this as the 'gender closet' and observes that this rhetoric obscures the way everyone is welcome online but only if they masquerade as the dominant group. Thus the rhetorical empowerment exists only when disability is erased. Just because the stereotypes are not projected onto a person does not mean they do not continue to exist. This belief also rests on a premise of passing as the correct and socially acceptable thing to do.

Conclusion

New media is increasingly providing the infrastructure through which to view and experience popular culture and the debates it elicits. Spreadable media leverages emotion to create viral content – people pass content from person to person through social networking sites at a rapid pace because it has somehow 'infected' them, like a virus. Spreadable media relies on people's intervention, their decisions to pass something on to their networks. Perhaps liking a Facebook page about a boy with Asperger's who does not have friends to invite to his birthday party fulfils some need in the liker, maybe it says something about the liker's worldview. Facebook is like the clothes we wear, we want it to tell people what we are like, where we fit in.

We might call this slacktivism, a simulacra of activism without actually having to do anything or change beliefs and behaviours, let alone the structure of society itself. However, online spreadable media can offer an alternative to media power which has been shown to be damaging towards public perception of people with disability. Additionally, online discourse offers disability more media attention and allows people with disability a voice in debates from which they are usually excluded. This, according to Lévy, is how knowledge can be advanced through collective intelligence.

However, discourses of disability associated with charity, inspiration and existential guilt continue to dominate online as the social spam of the twenty-first century. This chapter has also offered a history of sorts of disability in new media as popular culture – from disability blogging to participating in social media, to controlling the mode of production in Teal Sherer's web series *My Gimpy Life*. Again, disability features in every aspect of online media. However, among this celebration we must remain constantly aware of the inaccessibility and discriminatory attitudes that continues to pervade the web.

Chapter 9

Conclusion:
Focusing Passion, Creating
Community, Expressing Defiance

'Blue Ear' is a superhero in the *Marvel* comic book universe whose hearing aids help him hear when 'someone is in trouble'. The character was inspired by Anthony Smith, a four-year-old with hearing impairments who stopped wearing his hearing aids to school in 2012. When he complained to his mother that none of his favourite comic book superheroes needed to wear blue ears, she emailed *Marvel* comics who sent her a comic book cover from the 1980s featuring Hawkeye, a member of the Avengers who wore hearing aids and continued his crime fighting duties when he lost 80% of his hearing. Nelson Ribeiro, an artist at *Marvel*, then set about developing the concept of Blue Ear, a crime fighting superhero who used his 'listening devices' to '[listen] for people in trouble and he goes to help them and he fights bad guys' (Anthony Smith cited in Hanson, 2012).

This might seem like a bit of fun – a cute story about a kid, comic books and superheroes – but hearing aids are a controversial example with critical disability studies. Numerous critiques surround cochlear implants, cultures of compulsory correction, and the propensity to present people with disability as heroic for simply living their lives. However, I use this example to illustrate the importance of popular culture in addressing the social inclusion of people with disability and for proving opportunities for identification and discussion.

Throughout this book I have attempted to take a producerly approach to disability in popular culture. It has been my goal to question why the social and cultural models of disability have not been able to address the pleasures people gain from engaging with popular culture, or indeed considered the reality that popular culture changes, that it moves with the times, that shifting values and attitudes regarding disability can be discerned even in popular culture mass-produced within a capitalist system, that popular culture is political. Indeed disability in popular culture can offer an accessible way to explain key points in critical disability studies.

While taking this optimistic approach to disability and popular culture, I also argue that there is a great deal of work left to do in this area, and that questioning current representations and instances of disability in popular

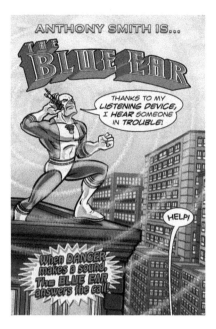

Figure 9.1 *The Blue Ear*

Source: © 2014 MARVEL.

culture is vitally important. Yet, as I have discussed throughout this book, despite the progress made, disability in popular culture is frequently interpreted through a patronising lens, particularly by the media. For example, the children's toys discussed in Chapter 2 such as Share a Smile Becky, the Hal's Pals or even Melissa Yang's request for an American Doll with a disability are viewed as considerate deeds for the 'poor disabled' who are 'not like us'. Similarly, the movies, athletes and television programs discussed in chapters 4, 5 and 7 are invariably described as inspirational, a paradigm that maintains the pitiable discourse that social and cultural models of disability have sought to expose as more condescending than empowering. As Dan Goodley (2011) argues, 'to be disabled evokes a marginalised place in society, culture, economics and politics' (p. 1). He identifies a cultural redefinition of disability emerging through a so-called minority model of disability that recognises that 'PWD comprise a minority group that has been denied its civil rights, equal access and protection' (p. 14).

Snyder and Mitchell (2006) locate this denial through cultural dis-locations such as eugenics that have established the social and cultural view that people with disabilities are biologically deviant. They explain that a 'cultural model' of disability exists in the space between embodiment and social ideology (p. 10). Making comparisons to the social model of disability – which has focused almost exclusively on social ideology or disability as the socially created restriction of activity imposed on top of people who have impairments – a cultural mode prioritises identity politics and recognises the way disability is created at the level of discourse. Thus, disability which has a material reality is also shaped by cultures.

Social and cultural critiques of disability often proceed from the notion that popular culture is more interested in making us feel, than in making us think, and that stereotypical and limiting discourses of disability are implicated in this process. Theorists have been especially critical of the way impairment is used in popular culture and the media to evoke an emotional response of fear in the audience (see Barnes, Mercer, and Shakespeare, 1999). However, as Henry Jenkins (2007) explains, emotion is the defining characteristic of whether a piece of popular culture is considered a success. Jenkins argues that 'popular culture, at its best, makes us think by making us feel' (p. 3). For popular culture to succeed in making us think, Jenkins maintains, an incorporation of and experimentation with what has come before is crucial.

However, popular culture is constantly changing, constantly rearranging itself to entice our interest. While everything is derivative, these references take on new forms and new texts are created. These new texts offer a space for critical engagement and new images of disability. Although there is still much work to do, images in popular culture change to reflect changes in the social position of people with disability. In this concluding chapter, I seek to bring together the social and cultural models of disability to point to a new wave in disability criticism that recognises the ways people poach certain aspects of popular culture, use popular culture to make social critiques more visible, and gain pleasure from popular culture.

Throughout this book I have drawn on core ideas of both the social and cultural models of disability to urge critical disability theorists to look again at the importance of popular culture to people's sense of selves and identity formation as people with disability. In line with social model critiques, I have argued that popular culture does contribute to and reflect the disablement of people with disability, and that it is vital to increase the employment of people with disability in the cultural industries. Secondly, I agree with cultural models of disability which argue that popular culture establishes boundaries of normality and is influenced by other institutions and establishments.

The social model of disability has been effective in raising awareness of the disempowerment experienced through disabling responses to impairments, while the cultural models consider the ways disability oppression of particular eras has been reflected in the narratives created and the tendency of cultural narratives to demarcate the boundary between who is considered human and who is not. However, neither model has adequately explained the pleasure people gain from popular culture, and the use it has in their lives to mark out a proud disability identity and community. Both models have pointed towards avant-garde disability cultural production as the way forwards to challenge disability social oppression and force an ableist world to interrogate their prejudicial beliefs. The cultural production that they encourage could be described as writerly. While this is a vital area for critical disability studies to explore, this book has focused instead on popular culture. Those readerly texts that, through popular consumption, become producerly. As John Fiske (1989, 2010) argues in *Understanding Popular Culture*, popular culture, although produced 'under conditions of social subordination', is 'always, at its heart, political' (p. 126).

I began this book with Steve Tucker's email attempt to locate a woman he met in a bar and the impacts his coming out as disabled had on the way the story was reported and indeed the public's reaction to it. Two years before Tucker's email went viral and he became the latest Romeo of spreadable media, *Breaking Bad* premiered on American television. Protagonist and antihero Walter White was the consequence of a life of regrets that Tucker wrote about. Walter began in season 1 as the everyman working hard to ensure his family's future. Working two thankless jobs (as a high school chemistry teacher during the day and in a car wash at night), routinely humiliated by his students at work and brother-in-law Hank at home, subject to the whims of his dominating pregnant wife and father to a teenager with cerebral palsy, Walter was heavy with 'regret' (Barnes, 2008). Actor Bryan Cranston described his character when the critically and popularly acclaimed series began as:

> ... a high school Chemistry [teacher], mid-life. Probably living in quiet desperation, with the weight of regret on his chest, and he probably didn't pursue the things he wanted to earlier in life and now he's faced with this midlife crisis. On top of that he finds out that he has terminal lung cancer and has one to two years to live. So he's having a bad day. At first he's numbed by that information and he doesn't know what to do with that. Then he realizes that he's about to go through this transformation in his body, and a deterioration, and at the end of it he's going to die. And his wife is going to care for him all the way and on top of that, he's going to leave them penniless. It's not as if he has any money to speak of now ... So in that desperate set of circumstances he decides to make a desperate move and that is to use his Chemistry background to make as much money as he possibly can before he dies, by cooking crystal meth and becoming a drug dealer. (Cranston cited in Barnes, 2008)

Walt's cancer diagnosis and son with cerebral palsy were narrative devices designed to ensure a sympathetic audience interpretation of a character who is essentially despicable. However, as *Breaking Bad* progressed, Walt changed, Walt Jnr changed, and the show became a fascinating exploration of illness, impairment and disabling social attitudes. Instead of being the inspirational cancer patient so frequently seen in popular culture, Walt became Heisenberg, the quick- and creative-thinking, murderous drug lord:

> ... you clearly don't know who you're talking to, so let me clue you in. I am not in danger, Skyler. I am the danger. A guy opens his door and gets shot and you think that of me? No. I am the one who knocks! (episode 6, season 4)

Breaking Bad is also notable for hiring R.J. Mitte, an actor with disability, to portray Walt Jnr. Initially designed as a narrative device to elicit audience sympathy for Walt, as the series progressed, Walt Jnr's disability was rarely emphasised. Despite this, the social inclusion of people with disabilities is drawn into the narrative several times across the trajectory of five seasons. For example, whereas in season 1 Walt admonishes his son for not driving a car the correct way, by season 4 Walt Jnr has convinced him of the suitability of his alternative driving accommodations. These minor narrative moments offer important disability critiques and reflect Walt's own shifting personality from a by-the-book chemistry teacher to the character of Heisenberg who lives by his own rules.

Disability is central to *Breaking Bad*'s questioning of social acceptability and why we behave the way we do when it may not be in our own best interests. Walt Jnr's producerly disability critiques are also integral to Hank's acceptance of his own disabling injury in seasons 3 and 4. Following a drug cartel assassination attempt against him, disability and impairment is depicted in a totally innovative way through Hank. As Hank becomes increasingly belligerent, Walt Jnr provides a voice of reason. When Hank refuses to return home unless he is walking, Walt Jnr asks him if people who use crutches (i.e. himself) should stay out of public view too. Haider Javed Warraich (2013) described *Breaking Bad* as the best medical drama on television. Instead of introducing a miraculous cure and smooth readjustment to life, Hank is shown throughout season 4 wallowing in self-pity, as he abuses loved ones, watches pornography, and amasses an enormous collection of 'minerals' purchased off the internet.

This book is interested in the Steve Tuckers, the Walter Whites, the Walt Jnrs and the Hanks – what we think of them, how we incorporate their stories into our lives, how the media interprets them and the ways they introduce important disability debates and reflect actual changes in the social position of people with disability.

Popular culture is a site of both resistance *and* incorporation. Unequal divisions between groups are both established and contested in popular culture, which then becomes an 'arena of struggle and negotiation between the interests of dominant groups and the interests of subordinate groups' (Storey, 2003, p. 51). People with disabilities are one such subordinate group and we can see moments of resistance in the way disability figures in popular culture.

The Popular Is Political

Throughout this book I've attempted to take an approach to disability and popular culture that goes beyond analysis of the assaults certain narratives have made on the lives of people with disability to recognise the pleasures in popular culture. This is the third wave of disability cultural criticism. A disability movement first emerged in response to narrow ways of understanding disability and has undergone several stages. Paul Longmore's discussion of these phases parallels a changing image of disability in popular culture and avant-garde disability art:

> The first phase has been a quest for civil rights, for equal access and equal opportunity, for inclusion. The second phase is a quest for collective identity. Even as the unfinished work of the first phase continues, the task in the second phase is to explore or create a disability culture. (Longmore, 2003, p. 215)

Even as the unfinished work of the first and second phases identified by Longmore continue, a third phase, powered by people engaging with not just disability culture, but popular culture broadly, is offering new insights. While some of the texts discussed throughout this book may not fit into a strictly social model conception of what disability in popular culture should be, as I have argued, they offer very important critiques of social oppression and explore themes relevant to the disability experience.

Textual poaching is vital to this discussion and throughout this book I have considered poaching in its broadest sense. I have looked at examples of textual poaching which concentrate only on the progressive aspects of the text – such as discussions regarding *Game of Thrones*, *Avatar* and *Friday Night Lights*, as well as those which use problematic instances of disability in popular culture such as Share a Smile Becky (Chapter 2), Ellen Stohl posing for *Playboy* (Chapter 3), the *Push Girls* reality TV show (chapters 3 and 5), and inspirational memes of Oscar Pistorius (Chapter 8) – to open discussions around disability social justice and offer opinions on the continuing subjugation of disability. Some case studies – such as Lady Gaga, discussed in Chapter 6 and the *Push Girls* discussed in Chapter 5 – have attracted both types of poaching.

As I discussed in Chapter 1, representations of disability in *Star Trek* have changed with the times – for example, whereas the Captain Pike of the 1960s was an object of pity and revulsion to his protégé Captain Kirk, 2009's Pike was more heroic, although continued to hand over control of his ship to the younger, more able, more masculine Kirk. While both representations have problematic aspects, how do we explain the ways audiences with disability describe the importance of *Star Trek* to their experience of disability and impairment?

I'm coming out as a disabled person (representing for fibromyalgia and chronic fatigue). I'm also coming out as a Trekkie. Believe it or not, the two things are connected, and not just because of all the Deep Space Nine I've watched while couchbound in a symptom flare-up. It was the belief of Star Trek creator Gene Roddenberry that, if humanity was to survive into the future, we would be required to not only tolerate differences between people and cultures but take special delight in them, celebrating them as one of the best parts of "life's exciting variety". It was a high calling then, in the era of the civil rights movement and early space exploration. It feels even loftier now. A wheelchair, a hearing aid, an inability to work full-time due to chronic illness: these are all examples of facets that differentiate people with disabilities from … the rest. The folks who can function within, shall we say, "normal parameters". (Henkelman, 2014)

Perhaps Henkleman is 'reading' disability themes into *Star Trek* or perhaps we could argue that a deeper understanding of disability enriches popular culture broadly. The popular culture discussed in this book, as with all popular culture, reveals the influence of aesthetics, technology, the quotidian and economics. This is revealed by looking at the features through a disability lens. Again, this can be seen in the long-running television program *Star Trek*. Over its original 4-year run, and later intergenerational iterations, *Star Trek* introduced a number of disabled bodies and technological advancements. Anthony Rotolo reflects on the ways students use *Star Trek* to engage with ideas related to society, humanity, technology and their own future possibilities:

> … a student who recalled how she had been captivated by the character of Geordi LaForge when first watching *The Next Generation* many years ago. As someone who was visually impaired herself, like the character of LaForge, she remembered marveling not only at the VISOR technology that allowed Geordi to see, but also that a person could so completely overcome blindness in the future. This student had found inspiration in that idea to pursue her own, successful career in science and technology. (Rotolo, 2014)

While this book has not been about science fiction specifically, I kept finding myself returning to the genre for the important debates it introduces around disability, minorities, inclusion, technology and the economy – science fiction themes emerged in my discussion of toys, beauty, movies, television, music video, sport and new media. I also found that even science fiction texts not specifically about disability can be enhanced through a disability lens of interpretation. For example, when Officer Alex J. Murphy is resurrected as the part-man part-machine cyborg Robocop after his body is obliterated by bad guys in Paul Verhoeven's cult movie *Robocop* (1987), his negotiation of the human body, technology and the wider socio-cultural environment illustrate debates about the rehabilitative promise of new technology for people with disability.

In the film, as a direct result of capitalist competition, the Robocop was created by the company Omni Consumer Products (OCP) as part of its corporate growth gamble in sectors traditionally regarded as non-profit. The company concentrated on technological change rather than the corresponding social change. OCP were unconcerned with the social impact beyond the profits they could reap from providing a mechanised service to decrease crime.

That Robocop was created out of a man with a broken body fits in with a rehabilitative discourse of disability deliverance through technology. As I have noted throughout this book, we are most familiar with individualised and medicalised discourses which suggests disability can be cured through medicine or technologies. While these technologies can compensate for impairment in a 'non-disabled' world, their cultural interpretation and relevance remains contested.

The film also explores disability as a social construction. Although theorists interested in this politicisation have accused technological development of contributing to the further disablement of people with impairments (Davis, 1995; Oliver, 1978), technology in a broad sense is integral to the politicisation of disability, particularly as we move further into an information age of both employment and leisure. *Robocop* can be considered under this radical perspective as the film forges links between technical and social change. The Robocop is welcomed into the force by the other police, uses technical supports to do his job, and is respected by the wider community. He does experience emotional and identity difficulties during his cyborg transition, however, which further highlight that technological advancement also involves a period of social adjustment.

As popular culture increasingly encounters digitisation, these science fiction themes become ever more important. I finished Chapter 8 with a brief discussion of disability access in the online environment. This is a vital discussion that actually impacts all of the instances of popular culture discussed in this book. For example, television is a leisure activity that many of us take for granted; however, it is beyond the reach of groups of people with disabilities for a number of reasons, including the effects of impairment, socio-economic status and technological development. As Joshua Robare (2011) explains, people with vision impairment are unable to enjoy television when video descriptions are not offered as a mainstream component of television programming. Yet, in the same way, people with a number of disabilities will benefit from accessibility options which promisingly are now becoming available as a result of digital television (see Utray, de Castro, Moreno, and Ruiz-Mezcua, 2012). Similarly, accessible toys, and especially games, are being developed, DVDs are beginning to include access features such as captions and audio description as a matter of course and accessibility features are introduced in mainstream Apple, Facebook, and Google products and platforms. This is a vital area of future research in an information age where access to leisure activity is increasingly recognised as equal in importance to access to the workforce, education and public space.

I have attempted to start a conversation in this book, a conversation I hope will continue in critical disability and popular culture studies. It is vital that further research takes place into audiences, publics and users. How do people with disability make meaning from popular culture and use it in their own lives to shape identity and community? A particularly important area of research is an interrogation of fan fiction and other user-generated content. Is disability recognised? Written into the narrative? Used as a narrative prosthesis? What happens when fans take responsibility for disability narratives? The future of critical disability studies relies on both academic and activist critique as well as a recognition of the way our concerns are reflected and critiqued in popular culture.

References

Abbasi, J. (2012, 16 July). Why 6-Year Old Girls Want to be Sexy. Retrieved 30 August, 2012, from http://www.livescience.com/21609-self-sexualization-young-girls.html

Abby jean. (2010a, 5 May). Psychiatric Hospitals and Music Videos: Part 1. Retrieved 23 August, 2013, from http://disabledfeminists.com/2010/05/05/psychiatric-hospitals-and-music-videos-part-1/

Abby jean. (2010b, 12 May). Psychiatric Hospitals and Music Videos: Part 2. Retrieved 23 August, 2013, from http://disabledfeminists.com/2010/05/05/psychiatric-hospitals-and-music-videos-part-1/

ABC news. (2013, 19 August). Lady Gaga 'Applause' Debut on 'GMA': 'Total Dream Come True'. Retrieved 24 August, 2013, from http://abcnews.go.com/blogs/entertainment/2013/08/lady-gaga-applause-debut-on-gma-total-dream-come-true/

Academic Editing Canada. (2013, 6 March). Blink Once for Yes: Remaking Disability in Star Trek. Retrieved 7 April, 2014, from http://www.academiceditingcanada.ca/blog/item/109-star-trek-proposals

Alary, B. (2012, 29 August). Tracing the Paralympic movement's 'freak show' roots. Retrieved 12 February, 2014, from http://news.ualberta.ca/newsarticles/2012/08/tracingtheparalympicmovementfreakshowroots#sthash.8Mm0X9uf.dpuf

Allan, K. (2013). *Disability in Science Fiction: Representations of Technology as Cure.* New York: Palgrave Macmillan.

American Girl. (2014). American Girl: Follow Your Inner Star. Retrieved 27 January, 2014, from http://store.americangirl.com/agshop/static/goty.jsp

Arjan. (2008, 30 November). Arjan Interviews Lady GaGa. Retrieved 25 August, 2013, from http://www.arjanwrites.com/arjanwrites/2008/11/arjan-interview-lady-gaga.html

Arnold, M. (2006). *Culture and Anarchy.* Oxford and New York: Oxford University Press.

Bainbridge, J. (2010). Fully articulated: The rise of the action figure and the changing face of 'children's' entertainment. *Journal of Media and Cultural Studies, 24*(6), 829–42. doi: 10.1080/10304312.2010.510592

Barnes, C. (1992). Disabling imagery and the media: An exploration of the principles for media representations of disabled people. http://www.leeds.ac.uk/disability-studies/archiveuk/Barnes/disabling%20imagery.pdf

Barnes, C. (1992). Images of Disability on Television. *Disability, Handicap & Society*, *7*(4), 385–7. doi: 10.1080/02674649266780481

Barnes, C. (1997). A legacy of oppression: A history of disability in Western culture. In L. Barton and M. Oliver (eds), *Disability Studies: Past Present and Future* (pp. 3–24). Leeds: The Disability Press.

Barnes, C., Mercer, G., and Shakespeare, T. (1999). *Exploring Disability: A Sociological Introduction*. Malden: Polity Press.

Barnes, W. (2008, 22 September). Interview: Breaking Bad Star and Emmy Winner Bryan Cranston. Retrieved 1 April, 2014 from http://screencrave.com/2008-09-22/interview-breaking-bad-star-bryan-cranston/

Barton, C., and Somerville, K. (2012). Play Things: Children's Racialized Mechanical Banks and Toys, 1880–1930. *International Journal of Historical Archaeology*, *16*(1), 47–85. doi: 10.1007/s10761-012-0169-y

Benkler, Y. (2006). *The Wealth of Networks How Social Production Transforms Markets and Freedom [Electronic book]*. Retrieved from http://www.eblib.com.au/

Berger, A.A. (1980). *Television as an Instrument of Terror*. New Brunswick, NJ: Transaction Publishers.

Berke, J. (2011, 28 August). Parenting – Barbie's Deaf Friends. Retrieved 4 December, 2013, from http://deafness.about.com/cs/parentingarticles/a/barbiefriends.htm

Bernardin, M. (2008, 2 April). Taking a moment for National Autism Awareness Day. Retrieved September 11, 2013, from http://popwatch.ew.com/2008/04/02/autistism-aware/

Bertling, C., and Schierl, T. (2008). Disabled Sport and its Relation to Contemporary Cultures of Presence and Aesthetics. *Sport in History*, *28*(1), 39–50. doi: 10.1080/17460260801889202

Bérubé, M. (2005). Disability and Narrative. *PMLA*, *120*(2), 568–76. doi: 10.2307/25486186

Bignell, J. (2000). "Get Ready For Action!": Reading Action Man Toys. In D. Jones and T. Watkins (eds), *A Necessary Fantasy?: The Heroic Figure in Children's Popular Culture* (pp. 231–50). New York: Garland Publishing.

Bogdan, R. (1990). *Freak Show: Presenting Human Oddities for Amusement and Profit*. Chicago: University of Chicago Press.

Brabazon, T. (2004). *From Revolution to Revelation: Generation X, Popular Memory, and Cultural Studies*. Aldershot: Ashgate.

Brabazon, T. (2006). *Playing on the Periphery: Sport, Identity and Memory*. New York: Routledge.

Brabazon, T., and Redhead, S. (2013). Baudrillard in Drag: Lady Gaga and the Accelerated Cycles of Pop. *Americana: The Journal of American Popular Culture (1900-present)*, *12*(2), http://www.americanpopularculture.com/journal/articles/fall_2013/brabazon_redhead.htm

Braidotti, R. (2010). On Putting the Active Back into Activism. *New Formations: A Journal of Culture/Theory/Politics, 68*, 42–57. doi: 10.3898/newf.68.03.2009

Brantlinger, P. (1991). Raymond Williams: 'Culture Is Ordinary'. *ARIEL: A Review of International English Literature, 22*(2), 75–81.

Brittain, I. (2013). *Disability Sport: A Vehicle For Social Change?* Champaign: Common Ground Publishing.

Bruns, A., and Jacobs, J. (2006). *Use of Blogs.* New York: Peter Lang.

Cafferty, D.D.R. (2012). *A Doll Like Me: Do Children with Down Syndrome Prefer to Play with Dolls That Have the Physical Features Associated with Down Syndrome?* (MS thesis), U of California.

Cain, M.C. (2010). Of pain, passing and longing for music. *Disability and Society, 25*(6), 747–51. doi: 10.1080/09687599.2010.505751

Calvert, D. (2013). 'A person with some sort of learning disability': the aetiological narrative and public construction of Susan Boyle. *Disability and Society*, 1–14. doi: 10.1080/09687599.2013.776484

Cameron, A. (2012). All we hear is Lady-o Gaga: Popular Culture 2.0. In T. Brabazon (ed.), *Digital Dialogues and Community 2.0: After Avatars, Trolls and Puppets* (pp. 209–18). Oxford: Chandos.

Cameron, C. (2009). Tragic but brave or just crips with chips? Songs and their lyrics in the Disability Arts Movement in Britain. *Popular Music, 3*, 381–96.

Campbell, F.K. (2011, 19 July). Born this Way? Lady Gaga's Crip Performance of the Wheelchair. Retrieved 24 August 2013, from http://www.griffith.edu.au/criminology-law/griffith-law-school/news-events/news/lady-gaga-crip-performance-wheelchair

Carlson, L.A. (2013). Wired for Interdependency: Push Girls and cyborg sexuality. *Feminist Media Studies, 13*(4), 754–9. doi: 10.1080/14680777.2013.805591

Carlson, T. (2012, 3 July). Push Girls Episode 6 review: Fired Up. Retrieved 25 April, 2014, from http://beautyability.com/about-3/

Carter, N., and Williams, J. (2012). 'A genuinely emotional week': learning disability, sport and television – notes on the Special Olympics GB National Summer Games 2009. *Media, Culture and Society, 34*(2), 211–27. doi: 10.1177/0163443711430759

Casablanca, T., and Weisman, A. (2011). News/Bette Midler to Lady Gaga: "Keep the Meat Dress and the Firecracker Tits. The Mermaid's Mine". Retrieved 24 August, 2013, from http://au.eonline.com/news/252813/bette-midler-to-lady-gaga-keep-the-meat-dress-and-the-firecracker-tits-the-mermaid-s-mine

CBCNews.Ca. (2014, 12 March). Sochi Paralympics: Corporate sponsorship the 'last barrier' for athletes. Retrieved 17 April, 2014, from https://ca.news.yahoo.com/corporate-sponsorship-last-barrier-paralympians-090000482.html

Celeb Daily News. (2013). Is Lady Gaga's 'ARTPOP' a total flop which will lose her label millions of dollars?. Retrieved 23 January, 2014, from http://

celebdailynews.com/is-lady-gagas-artpop-a-total-flop-which-will-lose-her-label-millions-of-dollars/

Ceramic teaching doll to show treatment for polio, England, 1930–1950. Retrieved 2 February, 2014, from http://www.sciencemuseum.org.uk/broughttolife/objects/display.aspx?id=5894

Channel 4 Press. (2010, 9 August). Two Years to Change Perception of Disability Sport. Retrieved 18 October, 2013, from http://www.channel4.com/info/press/news/two-years-to-change-perception-of-disability-sport

Chemers, M. (2005). Introduction Staging Stigma: A Freak Studies Manifesto *Disability Studies Quarterly*, *25*(3), http://dsq-sds.org/article/view/574/751

Cheyne, R. (2009). Introduction: Popular Genres and Disability Representation. *Journal of Literary & Cultural Disability Studies*, *6*(12), 117–23

Church, D. (2006). 'Welcome to the Atrocity Exhibition': Ian Curtis, Rock Death, and Disability *Disability Studies Quarterly*, *26*(4), http://dsq-sds.org/article/view/804/979

CIPR. (2012). Best Sporting Campaign – case study. Retrieved 12 February, 2014, from http://www.cipr.co.uk/content/events-awards/excellence-awards/results/5-best-sporting-campaign/case-study

Clogston, J. (1994). The Disabled, the media, and the information age/ edited by Jack A. Nelson. In J.A. Nelson (ed.), (pp. 45–57). Westport, CT: Greenwood Press.

Coach G. (2007, 20 March). Scott Porter of 'Friday Night Lights'. Retrieved 17 November, 2013, from http://featuresblogs.chicagotribune.com/entertainment_tv/2007/03/scott_porter.html

Cook, C. (2013, 19 August). Most memorable Reading Festival moments: Kurt Cobain comes on stage in a wheelchair in 1992. Retrieved 22 January, 2014, from http://www.getreading.co.uk/whats-on/music/most-memorable-reading-festival-moments-5750739

Cooper, C. (1995). Playboy interview: Hugh Hefner and Playmate Ellen Stohl Talk with Chet Cooper. Retrieved 5 March, 2014, from http://www.abilitymagazine.com/charles-Hugh%20Hefner-stohl.html

Corona, V.P. (2011). Memory, Monsters, and Lady Gaga. *The Journal of Popular Culture*, no-no. doi: 10.1111/j.1540-5931.2011.00809.x

Couldry, N., and Curran, J. (2003). *Contesting Media Power: Alternative Media in a Networked World.* Oxford: Rowman & Littlefield.

Courtney. (2009a, 1 October). Chivalry Doesn't Seem So Dead. Retrieved 27 February, 2014, from http://feministing.com/2009/10/01/chivalry-doesnt-seem-so-dead/

Courtney. (2009b, 28 October). Follow Up on Disability Rights Dialogue. Retrieved 21 February, 2014, from http://feministing.com/2009/10/28/follow-up-on-disability-rights-dialogue/comment-page-1/

Cox, D.R. (1977). Barbie and Her Playmates. *The Journal of Popular Culture, 11*(2), 303–7. doi: 10.1111/j.0022-3840.1977.00303.x

Cresswell, A. (2008, 12 July). Dolls with disabilities divide opinion. Retrieved 26 December, 2008, from http://www.theaustralian.news.com.au/story/0,25197,24000338-23289,00.html

Cumberbatch, G., and Negrine, R. (1992). *Images of Disability on Television.* London: Routledge.

Cummings, J. (1987, 8 June). Disabled Model Defies Sexual Stereotypes. Retrieved 7 March, 2014, from http://www.nytimes.com/1987/06/08/style/disabled-model-defies-sexual-stereotypes.html

Dan, O. (2010, 26 January). A Difference in Perspective: Experiencing Avatar Exceeds the Marketing. Retrieved 25 September, 2013, from http://disabledfeminists.com/2010/01/26/a-difference-in-perspective-experiencing-avatar-exceeds-the-marketing/

Danziger, L. (2009, 10 August). SELF speaks out about Kelly Clarkson photo retouching. Retrieved 13 March, 2014, from http://shine.yahoo.com/healthy-living/self-speaks-out-about-kelly-clarkson-photo-retouching-499107.html

Darke, P. (2004). The Changing Face of Representations of Disability in the Media. In J. Swain, S. French, C. Barnes and C. Thomas (eds), *Disabling Barriers – Enabling Environments* (pp. 100–105). Los Angeles: Sage.

Davis, L. (1995). *Enforcing Normalcy: Disability, Deafness, and the Body.* London: Verso.

Davis, L. (2005, 21 February). Why Disability Studies Matters. Retrieved 6 August, 2013, from http://www.insidehighered.com/views/2005/02/21/ldavis1

de Brito, S. (2010, 30 November). The real Steve Tucker story. Retrieved 31 March, 2014, from http://blogs.smh.com.au/executive-style/allmenareliars/2010/11/30/therealsteve.html

DePauw, K.P., and Gavron, S.J. (2005). *Disability Sport* (Second ed.). Champaign: Human Kinetics.

Deveney, C. (2013, 8 December). Susan Boyle: 'I have Asperger's'. Retrieved 3 March, 2014, from http://www.theguardian.com/fashion/2013/dec/08/susan-boyle-i-have-aspergers

Diament, M. (2010, 9 November). Max From NBC's 'Parenthood' Talks Asperger's. Retrieved 11 January, 2014, from http://www.disabilityscoop.com/2010/11/09/parenthood/11084/

Dictionary, O.E. *"invalid, adj.1"*: Oxford University Press.

Dictionary, O.E. *"invalid, adj.2 and n"*: Oxford University Press.

Diedrichs, P.C., and Lee, C. (2010). GI Joe or Average Joe? The impact of average-size and muscular male fashion models on men's and women's body image and advertisement effectiveness. *Body Image, 7*(3), 218–26. doi: 10.1016/j.bodyim.2010.03.004

Dilling-Hansen, L. (2012). A Bad Romance: Lady Gaga and the return of the divine monster. Retrieved 24 August, 2013, from http://www.inter-disciplinary.net/at-the-interface/wp-content/uploads/2012/08/DRAFTPAPERLiseDilling.pdf

Disability Bitch. (2008). Disability Bitch vs flat shoes. *Ouch! It's a Disability Thing*. Retrieved 26 June, 2010, from http://www.bbc.co.uk/ouch/opinion/b1tch/disability_bitch_vs_flat_shoes.shtml

Disability Horizons. (2013, 30 May). Toys with Disabilities and Why they Matter. Retrieved 9 February, 2014, from http://disabilityhorizons.com/2013/05/toys-with-disabilities-and-why-they-matter/

Dobuzinskis, A. (2009, 20 April). Susan Boyle breaks past 100 million online views. Retrieved 23 February, 2014, from http://blogs.reuters.com/fanfare/2009/04/20/susan-boyle-breaks-past-100-million-online-views/

du Cille, A. (1994). Dyes and Dolls: Multicultural Barbie and the Merchandising of Difference. *Differences*, *6*(1), 46–68.

Duncan, K., Goggin, G., and Newell, C. (2005). Don't talk about me ... like I'm not here: Disability in Australian national cinema. *Metro*, *146/147* 152–9.

Eco, U. (1987 [1969]). *Travels in Hyperreality*. London: Picador.

Ellis, K., and Goggin, G. (2015). *Disability and the Media*. New York: Palgrave Macmillan. Manuscript submitted for publication.

Ellis, K., and Kent, M. (2011). *Disability and New Media*. New York: Routledge.

ESD. (2014). All dolls are special, but these dolls have a little something Extra!. Retrieved 2 February, 2014, from http://extraspecialdolls.com/oscommerce2/catalog/index.php?index.php

Fabregat, M., Costa, M., and M.Romero. (2005). Adaptation of Traditional Toys and Games to New Technologies: New Products Generation. In J. Goldstein (ed.), *Toys, Games, and Media* (pp. 225–40). Hoboken: Taylor and Francis.

Faulkner, J. (2008, 26 June). Disability Dolls. *What Sorts of People?*. Retrieved 13 December (no longer available), 2009, from http://whatsortsofpeople.wordpress.com/2008/06/26/disability-dolls/

Finger, A. (1998, Jan/Feb). Invalids, de-generates, high-tech zombies & old-fashioned Hollywood cripples. Retrieved 16 September, 2013, from http://www.ragged-edge-mag.com/jan98/movie01.htm

Finkelstein, V. (1980). Attitudes and Disabled People: Issues For Discussion. *Disability Archive UK*. Retrieved 5 June, 2010, from http://www.leeds.ac.uk/disability-studies/archiveuk/finkelstein/attitudes.pdf

Finkelstein, V. (1981). Disability and the helper/helped relationship: A Historical View. *Disability Archive UK*. Retrieved 5 June, 2010, from http://www.leeds.ac.uk/disability-studies/archiveuk/finkelstein/Helper-Helped%20Relationship.pdf

Fiske, J. (1986). MTV: Post-Structural Post-Modern. *Journal of Communication Inquiry*, *10*(1), 74–9. doi: 10.1177/019685998601000110

Fiske, J. (1987, 2006). *Television Culture*. London and New York: Routledge.

Fiske, J. (1989, 2010). *Undersatanding Popular Culture*. New York: Routledge.

Fleming, D. (1996). *Powerplay: Toys as Popular Culture*. New York: Manchester University Press.

Frost, L. (1996). The Circassian Beauty and the Circassian Slave: Gender, Imperialism, and American Popular Entertainment In R. Garland-Thomson (ed.), *Freakery: Cultural Spectacles of the Extraordinary Body*. New York: New York University Press, pp. 248–64..

Gagapedia. (2010). The Monster Ball – Dialogue transcript. Retrieved 24 August, 2013, from http://ladygaga.wikia.com/wiki/The_Monster_Ball_-_Dialogue_transcript

Gagapedia. (no date). Yüyi the Mermaid. Retrieved 23 January, 2014, from http://ladygaga.wikia.com/wiki/Y%C3%BCyi_the_Mermaid

Garland-Thomson, R. (1995). Integrating Disability Studies into the Existing Curriculum: The Example of 'Women and Literature' at Howard University. *Radical Teacher, 47*, 15–21.

Garland-Thomson, R. (1996). *Freakery: Cultural Spectacles of the Extraordinary Body*. New York: New York University Press.

Garland-Thomson, R. (2001, 1 January). Re-Shaping, Re-Thinking, Re-Defining: Feminist Disability Studies. Retrieved 6 February, 2014, from http://www.thefreelibrary.com/Re-shaping,%20Re-thinking,%20Re-defining:%20Feminist%20Disability%20Studies.-a084377500

Garland-Thomson, R. (2002). The Politics of Staring: Visual Rhetorics of Disability in Popular Photography. In S. Snyder, B.J. Brueggmann and R. Garland-Thomson (eds), *Disability Studies: Enabling the Humanities* (pp. 56–85). New York: The Modern Language Association of America.

Garland-Thomson, R. (2004). Integrating disability: Transforming feminist theory. In B.G. Smith and B. Hutchison (eds), *Gendering Disability* (pp. 73–103). New Brunswick, N.J.: Rutgers University Press.

Garland-Thomson, R. (2006). Foreword. In N. Lerner and J. Straus (eds), *Sounding Off: Theorizing Disability in Music*. New York, London: Routledge.

Garland-Thomson, R. (2007). Shape structures story: fresh and fiesty stories about disability. *Narrative, 15*(1), 113–23.

Garland-Thomson, R. (2011). Integrating Disability, Transforming Feminist Theory. In K.Q. Hall (ed.), *Feminist Disability Studies*. Bloomington and Indianapolis: Indiana University Press.

Gerber, C. (2012, 17 February). Portrayals of the Disabled in Pop Culture. Retrieved 6 April, 2014, from http://disability.about.com/b/2012/02/17/portrayals-of-the-disabled-in-pop-culture.htm

Gerber, D. (1996). The "Careers" of People Exhibited in Freak Shows: The Problem of Violition and Valorization. In R.G. Thomson (ed.), *Freakery: The Cultural Spectacles of the Extraordinary Body* (pp. 38–54). New York: New York University Press.

GI Joe meets the Amazing Atomic Man!. Retrieved 7 February, 2014, from http://gijoe.wikia.com/wiki/GI_Joe_meets_the_Amazing_Atomic_Man!

Gilje, S. (1997, 7 June). Barbie's friend finds doors closed. Retrieved 4 December, 2013, from http://www.washington.edu/doit/Press/06.07.97.times.html

Giroux, H. (1998). Stealing Innocence: the Politics of Child Beauty Pagents. In H. Jenkins (ed.), *The Children's Culture Reader*. New York: New York University Press.

GLAAD (Gay and Lesbian Alliance Against Defamation). (2010). Where we are on tv. Retrieved from http://www.glaad.org/files/whereweareontv2010-2011.pdf

GLAAD (Gay and Lesbian Alliance Against Defamation). (2012). Where we are on TV 2012–2013. Retrieved from http://www.glaad.org/files/whereweareontv12.pdf

GLAAD (Gay and Lesbian Alliance Against Defamation). (2013). 2013 Where we are on TV. Retrieved 22 October, 2013, from http://www.glaad.org/files/2013WWATV.pdf

Goldmark, D. (2006). Stuttering in American Popular Song – 1890–130. In N. Lerner and J. Straus (eds), *Sounding Off: Theorizing Disability in Music* (pp. 91–105). New York and London: Routledge.

Goldstein, J. (2005). *Toys, Games, and Media*. Hoboken: Taylor and Francis.

Goodley, D. (2011). *Disability Studies: An Interdisciplinary Introduction*. Los Angeles: Sage.

Gray, J. (2008). *Television Entertainment*. New York: Routledge.

Gray, J. (2010). *Show Sold Separately: Promos, Spoilers, and Other Media Paratexts*. New York: New York University Press.

Gray, R.J. (2012). *The Performance Identities of Lady Gaga: Critical Essays*. Retrieved from http://CURTIN.eblib.com.au/patron/FullRecord.aspx?p=928856

Greene, B. (1987, 16 May). An Uncomfortable Issue For Playboy. Retrieved 30 March, 2014, from http://articles.chicagotribune.com/1987-05-17/features/8702060592_1_arthur-kretchmer-ellen-stohl-playboy

Grossberg, J. (2011, 14 July). News/Lady Gaga's Disabled Mermaid Wheelchair Bit Sparks Controversy … and Egg Attack?. Retrieved 24 August, 2013, from http://au.eonline.com/news/252298/lady-gaga-s-disabled-mermaid-wheelchair-bit-sparks-controversy-and-egg-attack

Gutierrez, P., and Martorell, A. (2011). People with intellectual disability and ICTs/Las personas con discapacidad intelectual ante las TIC.(RESEARCH). *Comunicar, 18 N 36*, 173.

Hall, K.J. (2004). A Soldier's Body: GI Joe, Hasbro's Great American Hero, and the Symptoms of Empire. *The Journal of Popular Culture, 38*(1), 34–54. doi: 10.1111/j.0022-3840.2004.00099.x

Hall, K.Q. (2011). *Feminist Disability Studies*. Bloomington, IN: Indiana University Press.

Hall, S. (1997). *Representation: Cultural Representations and Signifying Practices*. London: Sage Publications in association with the Open University.

Haller, B. (2000). If they limp, they lead? News representations and the hierarchy of disability images. In D. Braithwaite and T. Thompson (eds), *Handbook of Communication and People with Disabilities* (pp. 225–37). Mahwah, NJ: Lawrence Erlbaum.

Haller, B., and Ralph, S. (2006). Are Disability Images in Advertising Becoming Bold And Daring? An Analysis of Prominent Themes in US and UK Campaigns. *Disability Studies Quarterly*, *26*(3).

Hamilton, A. (2009, 20 November). The Transcontinental Disability Choir: Disabililty Chic? (Temporary) Disability in Lady Gaga's "Paparazzi". Retrieved 10 August, 2013, from http://bitchmagazine.org/post/the-transcontinental-disability-choir-disabililty-chic-temporary-disability-in-lady-gagas-papar

Hanson, J. (2012, 26 May). Superheroes do wear blue ears, thanks to NH boy. Retrieved 18 April, 2014, from http://www.unionleader.com/article/20120526/NEWS/705269948

Harris, L. (2002). Disabled Sex and the Movies. *Disability Studies Quarterly*, *22*(4), http://dsq-sds.org/article/view/378/503.

Hart, J. (2009). Video on the Internet: The Content Question. In D. Gerbarg (ed.), *Television Goes Digital* (pp. 131–45). New York: Springer.

Hartley, J. (2008). The twenty-first-century telescreen. In G. Turner and J. Tay (eds), *Television Studies After TV: Understanding Television in the Post-Broadcast Era*. London and New York: Routledge.

Hartley, J. (2010). *Digital Futures for Cultural and Media Studies*. Milton, Queensland: Wiley-Blackwell.

Headlam, D. (2006). Learning to Hear Autistically. In N. Lerner and J. Straus (eds), *Sounding Off: Theorizing Disability in Music*. New York, London: Routledge.

Henkelman, J. (2014, 2 March). Star Trek and disability. Retrieved 9 April, 2014, from http://www.geezmagazine.org/magazine/article/star-trek-and-disability/

Herr, C. (2009). Roll-over-Beethoven: Johnnie Ray in context. *Popular Music*, *28*(Special Issue 03), 323–40. doi: doi:10.1017/S0261143009990092

Hevey, D. (1992). *The Creatures Time Forgot: Photography and Disability Imagery*. London: Routledge.

Hiatt, B. (2009, 11 June). Lady Gaga, New York Doll. Retrieved 24 August, 2013, from http://www.rollingstone.com/music/news/lady-gaga-new-york-doll-rolling-stones-2009-cover-story-20090611

Hildebrand, J. (2013, 11 July). Exclusive: Kevin Rudd Hates Disabled People – The Incredible Proof Inside. Retrieved 5 October, 2013, from http://blogs.news.com.au/dailytelegraph/joehildebrand/index.php/dailytelegraph/comments/exclusive_kevin_rudd_hates_disabled_people_the_incredible_proof_inside/

Hollier, S. (2012). Sociability: Social Media for People with a Disability. Retrieved 31 May, 2013, from http://mediaaccess.org.au/online-media/social-media

Horkheimer, M., and Adorno, T.W. (1972). *Dialectic of Enlightenment* New York: Herder and Herder.

Hoyle, A. (2009, 16 August). The young student with a prosthetic arm who took on – and beat – a global fashion giant tells the full story of her humiliating ordeal. Retrieved 4 March, 2014, from http://www.dailymail.co.uk/femail/article-1206802/The-young-student-prosthetic-arm-took--beat--global-fashion-giant-tells-story-humiliating-ordeal.html#ixzz2arZt8V5S

Inquirer Wire Services. (1986, 4 June). Dolls With Disabilities Introduced By Mattel. Retrieved 8 December, 2013, from http://articles.philly.com/1986-06-04/entertainment/26043710_1_girl-with-leg-braces-hal-s-pals-disabled-children

International Paralympic Committee (IPC) (n.d). Football 5-a-side. Retrieved 12 February, 2014, from http://www.paralympic.org/football-5-side

IPC. (2014). Introduction to IPC Classifications. Retrieved 17 April, 2014, from http://www.paralympic.org/classification

Jenkins, H. (2007). *The Wow Climax: Tracing the Emotional Impact of Popular Culture.* New York and London: New York University Press.

Jenkins, H. (2013). *Spreadable Media: Creating Value and Meaning in a Networked Culture.* New York: New York University Press.

Jenkins, H., McPherson, T., and Shattuc, J. (2002). *Hop on Pop: The Politics and Pleasures of Popular Culture.* Durham, NC: Duke University Press.

johnboy. (2010, 16 November). Has anyone seen Olivia? Retrieved 31 March, 2014, from http://the-riotact.com/has-anyone-seen-olivia/31384

Johnson, C. (2002). De-gene-erates, Replicants and Other Aliens: (Re)defining Disability in Futuristic Film. In M. Corker and T. Shakespeare (eds), *Disability/Postmodernity* (pp. 198–212). London, New York: Continuum.

Johnson, T. (2012, 20 October). Meet the Real Princess in this Picture … Our Daughter Katie. Retrieved 30 April, 2014, from http://rootsofhealthyliving.com/our-daughter-katie/

Kama, A. (2004). Supercrips versus the pitiful handicapped: Reception of disabling images by disabled audience members. *Communications: The European Journal of Communication Research, 29*(4), 447–66.

Karr, A. (2014, 22 January). Nicola Formichetti Talks Diesel's Next Campaign. Retrieved 1 May, 2014, from http://www.wwd.com/media-news/fashion-memopad/reboot-redux-7385640?module=hp-media

Katz, E. (2009). The End of Television. In E. Katz and P. Scannell (eds), *The ANNALS of the American Academy of Political and Social Science* (Vol. 625, pp. 6–18). Thousand Oaks, CA: SAGE Publications.

Kriegal, L. (1987). The Cripple in Literature. In A. Gartner and T. Joe (eds), *Images of the Disabled, Disabling Images.* New York: Praeger.

Kumari Campbell, F. (2009). *Contours of Ableism: The Production of Disability and Ableness* New York: Palgrave Macmillan

Kuppers, P. (2007). The Wheelchair's Rhetoric: The Performance of Disability. *TDR: The Drama Review*, *51*(4), 80–88.

Kusler, V. (2012, 20 August). 'Push Girls': Exploiting Disabilities or Promoting Inclusion? Retrieved 14 March, 2014, from http://www.adiosbarbie.com/2012/08/push-girls-exploiting-disabilities-or-promoting-inclusion/#sthash.piP4FvJX.dpuf

Kuster, E. (2012, 14 June). Fearless 'Push Girl' Angela Rockwood: 'I Literally Just Push Through It All And Try To Stay Positive'. Retrieved 4 March, 2014, from http://www.huffingtonpost.com/2012/06/14/fearless-push-girl-angela-rockwood_n_1595278.html

Lady Gaga. (2013, 13 February). Facebook Post. Retrieved 10 August, 2013, from https://www.facebook.com/ladygaga/posts/10151520333149574

Laird, S. (2014, 5 February). Canadian Paralympics Ad Is a Powerful Reality Check. Retrieved 17 April, 2014, from http://mashable.com/2014/02/04/canadian-paralympics-ad-is-a-powerful-reality-check/

LaSpina, N. (1988, 2 October). DISABLED WOMAN: The Forging of a Proud Identity. Retrieved 21 March, 2014, from http://www.disabilityculture.org/course/keynote.htm

Leaver, T. (2013a). Joss Whedon, Dr Horrible and the Future of Web Media. *Popular Communication*, *11*(2), 160–73.

Leaver, T. (2013b). The Social Media Contradiction: Data Mining and Digital Death. *M/C Journal*, *16*(2), http://journal.media-culture.org.au/index.php/mcjournal/article/viewArticle/625

Lerner, N., and Straus, J.N. (2006). Introduction. In N. Lerner and J. Straus (eds), *Sounding Off: Theorizing Disability in Music*. New York, London: Routledge.

Lévy, P. (1997). *Collective Intelligence: Mankind's Emerging World in Cyberspace* (R. Bononno, trans.). New York and London: Plenum Press.

Liebowitz, C. (2010a, 15 December). Hey look, I'm hosting a blog carnival!!!. Retrieved 1 March, 2014, from http://thatcrazycrippledchick.blogspot.com.au/2010_12_01_archive.html

Liebowitz, C. (2010b, 16 November). Three strikes, yerrrrrrrr out!!!. Retrieved 1 March, 2014, from http://thatcrazycrippledchick.blogspot.com.au/2010_11_01_archive.html

Linton, S. (1998). *Claiming Disability: Knowledge and Identity*. New York and London: New York University Press.

Longmore, P. (1987). Screening Stereotypes: Images of Disabled People in Television and Motion Pictures. In A. Gartner and T. Joe (eds), *Images of the Disabled, Disabling Images* (pp. 65–78). New York: Praeger.

Longmore, P. (2003). *Why I Burned My Book: And Other Essays on Disability*. Philadelphia: Temple University Press.

Lubet, A. (2011). *Music, Disability, and Society*. Philadelphia: Temple University Press.

Lwin, M., and Phau, I. (2008). The role of existential guilt appeals in charitable advertisements. Marketing Insights: School of Marketing Working Paper Series: no. 200805, Curtin University of Technology, School of Marketing.

Magers, P. (2011, 21 June). Disabled Woman Looks Back At Posing Nude For Playboy, Challenging Stigmas. Retrieved 21 March, 2014, from http://losangeles.cbslocal.com/2011/06/21/disabled-woman-looks-back-at-posing-nude-for-playboy-challenging-stigmas/

Mallett, R. (2009). Choosing 'stereotypes': debating the efficacy of (British) disability-criticism. *Journal of Research in Special Educational Needs*, *9*(1), 4–11. doi: 10.1111/j.1471-3802.2009.01111.x

maraleia. (2012). Push Girls: They Just Happen to Tool Around in Wheelchairs. Retrieved 2 May, 2014, from http://forums.televisionwithoutpity.com/topic/3213773-push-girls-they-just-happen-to-tool-around-in-wheelchairs/

Martin, D. (1997). Disability Culture: Eager to Bite the Hands That Would Feed Them. *New York Times*. Retrieved from http://www.nytimes.com/1997/06/01/weekinreview/eager-to-bite-the-hands-that-would-feed-them.html?pagewanted=all

Mattel, I. (1997). Mattel Launches School Photographer Becky; Barbie Doll's Friend Who Uses A Wheelchair. Retrieved 4 December, 2013, from http://www.prnewswire.com/news-releases/mattel-launches-school-photographer-becky-barbie-dolls-friend-who-uses-a-wheelchair-75963267.html

McDonagh, R. (2013, 3 October). Rosaleen McDonagh pouts politics as she asks where disability representation in the media is heading?. Retrieved 14 March, 2014, from http://www.disabilityartsonline.org.uk/push-girls

McGowen, H.H. (2011, 1 March). Sensibilities, Self-Esteem and Shoes. Retrieved 31 March, 2014, from http://www.newmobility.com/2011/03/sensibilities-self-esteem-shoes/

McKay, G. (2013). *Shakin' All Over: Popular Music and Disability*. Ann Arbor: University of Michigan Press.

McKay, H. (2013, 4 June). 'Push Girls' reality stars seek to dispel the 'sloppy wheelchair stereotype'. Retrieved 18 March, 2014, from http://www.foxnews.com/entertainment/2013/06/03/push-girls-reality-stars-seek-to-dispel-sloppy-wheelchair-stereotype/

McKinley, E.G. (1997). *Beverly Hills, 90210: Television, Gender and Identity*. Philadelphia: University of Pennsylvania Press.

McReynolds, L. (2013). Animal and Alien Bodies as Prostheses: Reframing disability in Avatar and How to Train Your Dragon. In K. Allan (ed.), *Disability in Science Fiction: Representatioons of Technology as Cure*. New York: Palgrave Macmillan.

McRuer, R. (2006). *Crip Theory: Cultural Signs of Queerness and Disability*. New York and London: New York University Press.

Media Centre. (2012, 19 December). No. 13: Channel 4 creates a blueprint for commercial Paralympic broadcasting. Retrieved 18 October, 2013, from http://newsite.paralympic.org/feature/no-13-channel-4-creates-blueprint-commercial-paralympic-broadcasting

Michaels, S. (2013, 13 March). Lady Gaga using 24-carat gold wheelchair. *The Guardian.* Retrieved 10 August, 2013, from http://www.theguardian.com/music/2013/mar/13/lady-gaga-gold-wheelchair?CMP=twt_gu

Miller, C. (n.d.). J.J. Armes Action Figures – Turning Disability Into True Ability. Retrieved 7 February, 2014, from http://www.journalofantiques.com/April07/playing_around.html

Miller, T. (2001). *Sportsex.* Philadelphia: Temple University Press.

Miserandino, C. (2010). Dear Lady Gaga: a Love Letter from a Lupus Patient. Retrieved 24 August, 2013, from http://www.butyoudontlooksick.com/wpress/articles/written-by-christine/dear-lady-gaga-a-love-letter-from-a-lupus-patient/

Mitchell, D., and Snyder, S. (2000). *Narrative Prosthesis: Disability and the Dependencies of Discourse.* Ann Arbor: The University of Michigan Press.

Moody, N. (1997). Untapped Potential: The Representation of Disability/ Special Ability in the Cyberpunk Workforce. *Convergence: The International Journal of Research into New Media Technologies, 3*(3), 90–105. doi: 10.1177/135485659700300307

Moore, L. (2012, 21 August). "Push Girls" Needs to Push Back! By Guest Amoeblogger Leroy Moore. Retrieved 20 March, 2014, from http://www.amoeba.com/blog/2012/08/jamoeblog/-push-girls-needs-to-push-back-by-guest-amoeblogger-leroy-moore-.html

Morrison, E., and Finkelstein, V. (1997). Broken Arts and Cultural Repair: the role of culture in the empowerment of disabled people. In A. Pointon and C. Davis (eds), *Framed: Interrogating Disability in the Media* (pp. 160–65). London: British Film Institute.

Mr Magoo Toy Car, 1960s. Retrieved 4 December, 2013, from http://everybody.si.edu/media/749

Mueller, R. (n.d). Toy Catalogues. Retrieved 6 February, 2014, from http://antiquetoycollections.info/pages/catalogs.asp

Müller, F., Klijn, M., and Van Zoonen, L. (2012). Disability, prejudice and reality TV: Challenging disablism through media representations. *Telecommunications Journal of Australia, 62*(2), 28.21–8.13.

Multicultural Toys For Children of the '90s. (1995, 1 April). *Advertising Age*

Mulvey, L. (1975). Visual Pleasure and Narrative Cinema. *Screen, 16*(3), 6–18.

Naam, R. (2012). *More than Human: Embracing the promise of Biological Enhancement.* New York: Broadway Books.

Nachbar, J., and Lause, K. (1992). *Popular Culture: An Introductory Text.* Bowling Green: Bowling Green State University Popular Press.

Neale, S. (2000). *Genre and Hollywood.* London and New York: Routledge.

Neilsen, K. (2012). *A Disability History of the United States.* Boston: Beacon Press.

ngayonatkailanman. (2009, 13 April). Re: Susan Boyle Singing 'I Dreamed a Dream' from Les Miserables. [Online forum comment]. Retrieved from http://www.susan-boyle.com/messages/view/bckzxryvbfymd8qt

Noah's Ark. (2013). History. Retrieved 9 February, 2014, from http://www.noahsarkinc.org.au/who-are-we/histroy/

Norden, M. (1994). *The Cinema of Isolation: A History of Physical Disability in the Movies.* New Brunswick: Rutgers University Press.

O'Brien, K. (2005). *Warman's G.I. Joe Field Guide: Values and Identification.* Iola: Krause Publications.

Oliver, M. (1978). The misuse of Technology: walking appliances for paraplegics. *Journal of Medical Engineering & Technology, 2*(2), 69–70.

Oliver, M. (1990). *The Politics of Disablement.* Basingstoke, England: Macmillan Education.

Paglia, C. (2010, 12 September). Lady Gaga and the death of sex. Retrieved 24 August, 2013, from http://www.thesundaytimes.co.uk/sto/public/magazine/article389697.ece

Palmer, S. (2011). Old, New, Borrowed and Blue: Compulsory Able-bodiedness and Whiteness in Avatar. *Disability Studies Quarterly, 31*(1), http://dsq-sds.org/article/view/1353/1473.

Pearce, D. (2012, 22 October). All About Facebook 'Like' Scam Posts. Retrieved 23 February, 2014, from http://daylandoes.com/facebook-like-scams/

Peers, D. (2009). (Dis)empowering Paralympic histories: absent athletes and disabling discourses. *Disability & Society, 24*(5), 653–65. doi: 10.1080/09687590903011113

Penny, L. (2013). *Cybersexism: Sex, Gender and Power on the Internet.* London: Bloomsbury.

Person, L. (1998, October 9 1999). *Notes Toward a Postcyberpunk Manifesto.* Retrieved 7 September, 2013, from http://slashdot.org/story/99/10/08/2123255/notes-toward-a-postcyberpunk-manifesto

Phillips, L. (2012, 2 October). Viral Spam: Help a Human, Not a Hoaxer. Retrieved 23 February, 2014, from http://www.koozai.com/blog/social-media/facebook-social-media/viral-spam-help-a-human-not-a-hoaxer/

Pidd, H. (2009). Disabled student sues Abercrombie & Fitch for discrimination. *The Guardian.* Retrieved 23 November, 2012, from http://www.guardian.co.uk/money/2009/jun/24/abercrombie-fitch-tribunal-riam-dean

Pierce, B. (1997). Let the Old Creep Die. Retrieved 8 October, 2014, from https://nfb.org/images/nfb/publications/bm/bm97/bm971001.htm.

Pro Infirmus. (2013, 13 December). Because Who Is Perfect?. Retrieved 20 March, 2014, from https://www.youtube.com/watch?v=E8umFV69fNg

Quinlan, M., and Bates, B. (2008). Dances and Discourses of (Dis)Ability: Heather Mills's Embodiment of Disability on Dancing with the Stars. *Text and Performance Quarterly*, *28*(1–2), 64–80.

Quinlan, M.M., and Bates, B.R. (2009). Bionic Woman (2007): gender, disability and cyborgs. *Journal of Research in Special Educational Needs*, *9*(1), 48–58. doi: 10.1111/j.1471-3802.2009.01115.x

Reilly, J. (2012, 20 March). Glitter and grace: One-armed pole dancer impresses judges at world championships. Retrieved 21 September, 2013, from http://www.dailymail.co.uk/news/article-2117649/Deborah-Roach-armed-pole-dancer-crowned-winner-International-Championship.html#ixzz2arZHgf4o

Richards, P.L. (2012, 29 October). Disability Blog Carnival #84 is up NOW! Retrieved 1 March, 2014, from http://disstud.blogspot.com.au/2012/10/disability-blog-carnival-84-is-up-now.html

Richardson, N. (2010). *Transgressive Bodies: Representations in Film and Popular Culture*. Farnham: Ashgate.

Riddell, S., and Watson, N. (2003). *Disability, Culture, Identity*. Harlow: Pearson Education Limited.

Riley, C. (2005). *Disability and the Media: Prescriptions for Change*. Lebanon, NH: University Press of New England.

Robare, J.S. (2011). Television for All: Increasing Television Accessibility for the Visually Impaired Through the FCC's Ability to Regulate Video Description Technology. *Federal Communications Law Journal*, *63*(2), 553–78.

Robonut. (n.d.). Mike Power Atomic Man 1975 G.I.Joe. Retrieved 8 February, 2014, from http://www.robotnut.com/action/a1.htm

Rogers, M.F. (1999). *Barbie Culture*. London and Thousand Oaks, CA: SAGE Publications.

Roman Reed Foundation. (2011, 11 July). Tweet. Retrieved 24 August, 2013.

Rosenfeld, K.N. (2010). Terminator to Avatar: a postmodern shift. *Jump Cut: A Review of Contemporary Media*, *52*(Summer). Retrieved 8 October 2014 from http://www.ejumpcut.org/archive/jc52.2010/RosenfeldAvatar/text.html

Ross, K. (1997). But where's me in it? Disability, broadcasting and the audience. *Media, Culture & Society*, *19*(4), 669–77.

Rotolo, A. (2014, 20 January). TREK CLASS: Future Vision – The Tech of Trek. Retrieved 30 April, 2014, from http://www.startrek.com/article/trek-class-future-vision-the-tech-of-trek

Rowe, D. (1995). *Popular Cultures: Rock Music, Sport and the Politics of Pleasure*. London: Sage Publications.

s.e. smith. (2009, 1 October). An Open Letter to Feministing. Retrieved 21 February, 2014, from http://meloukhia.net/2009/10/an_open_letter_to_feministing/

Saito, S., and Ishiyama, R. (2005). The invisible minority: under-representation of people with disabilities in prime-time TV dramas in Japan. *Disability & Society, 20*(4), 437–51. doi: 10.1080/09687590500086591

Sandahl, C., and Auslander, P. (2005). *Bodies in Commotion: Disability & Performance.* Ann Arbor: University of Michigan Press.

Schell, L.A., and Duncan, M. (1999). A Content Analysis of CBS's Coverage of the 1996 Paralympic Games. *Adapted Physical Activity Quarterly, 16*, 27–47.

Schneider, S. (2009). *Science Fiction and Philosophy: From Time Travel to Superintelligence.* West Sussex: Wiley-Blackwell.

Schriempf, A. (2001). (Re)fusing the Amputated Body: An Interactionist Bridge for Feminism and Disability. *Hypatia, 16*(4), 53–79.

Scope. (2012). Superhuman or super athletes?. Retrieved 18 October, 2013, from http://www.scope.org.uk/news/disability-2012/superhuman-or-super-athletes

Seiter, E. (1995). *Sold Separately: Children and Parents in Consumer Culture.* New Brunswick, NJ: Rutgers University Press.

Sepinwall, A. (2012). *The Revolution was Televised: The Cops, Crooks, Slingers and Slayers Who Changed TV Drama Forever.* Austin, TX: Touchstone.

Shakespeare, T. (1999). Art and lies? Representations of disability on film. In M. Corker and S. French (eds), *Disability Discourse* (pp. 164–72). Buckingham: Open University Press.

Shakespeare, T. (2000, July). Disabled Sexuality: Towards Rights and Recognition. Retrieved 1 April, 2014, from http://bentvoices.org/culturecrash/shakespeare.htm

Shakespeare, T. (2006). *Disability Rights and Wrongs.* New York: Routledge.

Shang, M., and Shang, Y. (2014). American Girl: Release an American Girl with a disability. Retrieved 26 January, 2014, from http://www.change.org/petitions/american-girl-release-an-american-girl-with-a-disability

Shaw, M. (2010, 02 June). 'The Specials' Shows Life with Special Needs, Especially Watchable. Retrieved 30 November, 2012, from http://www.tubefilter.com/2010/06/02/the-specials-shows-life-with-special-needs-especially-watchable/

Shirky, C. (2008). *Here Comes Everybody: the Power of Organizing Without Organizations.* New York: Penguin Press.

Siebers, T. (2008). *Disability Theory.* Ann Arbor: University of Michigan Press.

Silva, C.F., and Howe, P.D. (2012). The (In)validity of Supercrip Representation of Paralympian Athletes. *Journal of Sport & Social Issues, 36*(2), 174–94. doi: 10.1177/0193723511433865

Smith, A., and Aaker, J. (2010). *The Dragonfly Effect: Quick, Effective and Powerful ways to use Social Media for Social Change.* Jossey-Bass: a Wiley Imprint.

Smith, L. (1988, 17 March). The Spirit of Ellen Stohl: Paralysis Doesn't Impair Her Fight for Human, Sexual Rights of Disabled – or Keep Her From

Posing for Playboy Layout. Retrieved 21 March, 2014, from http://articles. latimes.com/1988-03-17/news/li-1915_1_ellen-stohl

Snyder, S., and Mitchell, D. (2000). *Narrative Prosthesis: Disability and the Dependencies of Discourse.* Ann Arbor: The University of Michigan Press.

Snyder, S., and Mitchell, D. (2006). *Cultural Locations of Disability.* Chicago: The University of Chicago Press.

Snyder, S., and Mitchell, D. (2010). Body genres: An anatomy of disability in film. In S. Chivers and N. Markotić (eds), *The Problem Body: Projecting Disability on Film* (pp. 179–206). Columbus: The Ohio State University Press.

Sparrow, B. (2014, 12 February). Bec: This Woman is More than Brave. Retrieved 22 March, 2014, from http://www.mamamia.com.au/news/double-mastectomy-photos-beth-whaanga/

Stein, M.A. (1994). Mommy Has a Blue Wheelchair: Recognizing the parental rights of individuals with disabilities. *Brooklyn Law Review, 60,* 1069–693.

Stewart, D. (2013, 3 December). People With Disabilities React to Mannequins Created in Their Image. Retrieved 5 March, 2014, from http://jezebel.com/people-with-disabilities-react-to-mannequins-created-in-1475812519

Stokes, D. (2008). Blogging For Beginners. *Learning Disability Practice, 11*(3), 16–18.

Storey, J. (2003). *Inventing Popular Culture: From Folklore to Globalization.* Malden: Blackwell Publishing.

Straus, J. (2011). *Extraordinary Measures: Disability in Music.* Oxford: Oxford University Press.

Swartz, L., and Watermeyer, B. (2008). Cyborg anxiety: Oscar Pistorius and the boundaries of what it means to be human. *Disability & Society, 23*(2), 187–90. doi: 10.1080/09687590701841232

The Goldfish. (2010, 17 November). The Big Society and The Charity Model of Disability. Retrieved 1 March, 2014, from http://blobolobolob.blogspot.com.au/2010/11/big-society-and-charity-model-of.html

The Smoking Gun. (2006). ABC's 'Extreme' Exploitation: Makeover show loves sick kids, cancer patients, hate crime victims. Retrieved 2 May, 2014, from http://www.thesmokinggun.com/file/abcs-extreme-exploitation?page=0

The Sociological Cinema. (2014, 17 January). Building Manichean Bodies: The Problem with Those "Disabled" Mannequins. Retrieved 5 March, 2014, from http://www.thesociologicalcinema.com/1/post/2014/01/building-manichean-bodies-the-problem-with-those-disabled-mannequins.html#sthash.7aLJOLi7.dpuf

Thomas, C. (1999). *Female Forms: Experiencing and Understanding Disability.* Buckingham: Open University Press.

Thomas, N. (2008). *Disability Sport.* Hoboken: Taylor and Francis.

Thomas, N., and Smith, A. (2003). Preoccupied with Able-Bodiedness? An Analysis of the British Media Coverage of the 2000 Paralympics Games. *Adapted Physical Activity Quarterly, 20,* 166–81.

Thoreau, E. (2006). Ouch!: An Examination of the Self-Representation of Disabled People on the Internet. *Journal of Computer-Mediated Communication*, *11*(2), http://jcmc.indiana.edu/vol11/issue12/thoreau.html.

THR Staff. (2012, 5 June). Push Girls: TV Review. Retrieved 14 March, 2014, from http://www.hollywoodreporter.com/review/push-girls-tv-review-333331

Timberlake, C. (1986, 4 June). Hal's Pals May Have Very Limited Appeal, Toy Analyst Says. Retrieved 8 December, 2013, from http://www.apnewsarchive.com/1986/Hal-s-Pals-May-Have-Very-Limited-Appeal-Toy-Analyst-Says/id-adb38ba1986fd9e51ffc8241f4190aef

tmeronek. (2010, 10 August). Wheelchair Becky, Friend of Barbie. Retrieved 5 December, 2013, from http://whereslulu.com/2010/08/18/wheelchair-becky-friend-of-barbie/comment-page-1/#comment-246

Toffoletti, K. (2007). *Cyborgs and Barbie Dolls: Feminism, Popular Culture and the Posthuman Body*. London New York: I.B. Tauris.

Toys "R" Us. (2014). Toy Guide For Differently Abled Kids. Retrieved 9 February, 2014, from http://www.toysrus.com/shop/index.jsp?categoryId=3261680

Turner, G. (2009). *Ordinary People and the Media: the Demotic Turn*. London: SAGE.

Tusler, A. (2005). Don't Forget Who's Taking You Home. Retrieved 24 August, 2013 from http://www.e-bility.com/articles/disability-songs.php

Utray, F., de Castro, M., Moreno, L., and Ruiz-Mezcua, B. e. (2012). Monitoring Accessibility Services in Digital Television. *International Journal of Digital Multimedia Broadcasting*, *2012*, 9. doi: 10.1155/2012/294219

van Hilvoorde, I., and Landeweerd, L. (2008). Disability or Extraordinary Talent – Francesco Lentini (Three Legs) Versus Oscar Pistorius (No Legs). *Sport, Ethics and Philosophy*, *2*(2), 97–111. doi: 10.1080/17511320802221778

Velasquez, L. (2007). Downi Creations. Retrieved 4 December, 2009, from http://cause-of-our-joy.blogspot.com/2007/08/downi-creations.html

Vliet, P. v. d. (2012, 29 August). Paralympics 2012: Games classification system seeks to ensure that disability is no barrier to a level playing field. Retrieved 14 February, 2014, from http://www.telegraph.co.uk/sport/olympics/paralympic-sport/9506921/Paralympics-2012-Games-classification-system-seeks-to-ensure-that-disability-is-no-barrier-to-a-level-playing-field.html

Wade, L. (2010, 22 January). Lady Gaga's Disability Project. from http://thesocietypages.org/socimages/2010/01/22/lady-gagas-disability-project/

Walsh, T. (2005). *Timeless Toys: Classic Toys and the Playmakers Who Created Them*. Kansas City: Andrews McMeel.

Waltz, M., and James, M. (2009). The (re)marketing of disability in pop: Ian Curtis and Joy Division. *Popular Music*, *28*(3), 367–80.

Warraich, H.J. (2013, 10 September). Breaking Bad Is TV's Best Medical Drama, Ever. Retrieved 4 April, 42014, from http://www.slate.com/articles/health_and_science/medical_examiner/2013/09/breaking_bad_accuracy_a_doctor_says_it_s_the_best_medical_drama_on_tv.html

Was this woman's heartfelt facebook post really offensive? (2014, 12 February). Retrieved 31 March, 2014, from http://www.news.com.au/lifestyle/real-life/was-this-womans-heartfelt-facebook-post-really-offensive/story-fnixwvgh-1226824485413

Weihenmayer, E. (2008, May 12). Oscar Pistorius. Retrieved 2 August, 2013, from http://www.time.com/time/specials/2007/article/0,28804,1733748_1733756_1735285,00.html

Wendell, S. (1996). *The Rejected Body: Feminist Philosophical Reflections on Disability.* London and New York: Routledge.

Wheeler, T. (n.d.). Flashback Review: Mike Power – Atomic Man. Retrieved 7 February, 2014, from https://www.mastercollector.com/articles/reviews/review061105-3.htm

White, P. (2013). The triumph of hope over reality. Retrieved 18 October, 2013, from http://disabilitynow.org.uk/article/triumph-hope-over-reality

White Sidell, M. (2014, 24 January 2014). 'Its much more important than just an ad': Meet the wheelchair-bound star of Diesel's new campaign. Retrieved 13 March, 2014, from http://www.dailymail.co.uk/femail/article-2544271/Its-important-just-ad-Meet-wheelchair-bound-star-Diesels-new-campaign.html

Wickman, K. (2007). 'I do not compete in disability': How wheelchair athletes challenge the discourse of able-ism through action and resistance *European Journal for Sport and Society*, *4*(2), 151–67

Wilde, A. (2004). Are you sitting comfortably? Soap operas, disability and audience. *Dis: cover! 2.* Retrieved 18 June 2013, from. http://disability-studies.leeds.ac.uk/files/library/wilde-Alison-Wilde-Dis-cover-2-Adapted-Paper.pdf

Wilde, A., and Williams, D. (2011). Big Brother's Disabled Brother. *Celebrity Studies*, *2*(2), 224–6.

Wilkinson, D.Y. (1987). The Doll Exhibit: A Psycho-Cultural Analysis of Black Female Role Stereotypes. *The Journal of Popular Culture*, *21*(2), 19–30. doi: 10.1111/j.0022-3840.1987.2102_19.x

Willig Levy, C. (1998). A People's History of the Independent Living Movement. Retrieved 30 March, 2014, from http://www.independentliving.org/docs5/ILhistory.html#anchorContents

Willitts, P. (2012, 1 August). Bad attitudes do not cause disability any more than good attitudes guarantee health. Retrieved 25 February, 2014, from http://blogs.independent.co.uk/2012/08/01/bad-attitudes-do-not-cause-disability-any-more-than-good-attitudes-guarantee-health/

Wilson, E. (2003). *Adorned in Dreams: Fashion and Modernity.* London: I.B.Tauris.

Wilson, N. (2005). Excessive performances of the same: Beauty as the beast of reality TV. *Women & Performance: A Journal of Feminist Theory*, *15*(2), 207–29. doi: 10.1080/07407700508571512

Winter Is Coming. (2013, 22 October). Game of Thrones wins award honoring disability awareness. Retrieved 6 April, 2014, from http://winteriscoming. net/2013/10/game-of-thrones-wins-award-honoring-disability-awareness/

Wolf, N. (1993). *The Beauty Myth.* London: Vintage.

Wolf, N. (2002). *The Beauty Myth: How Images of Beauty are Used against Women.* New York: Harper Collins.

Young, S. (2011, 15 July). Going Gaga over wheels. Retrieved 12 January, 2014, from http://www.abc.net.au/rampup/articles/2011/07/15/3270307.htm

Young, S. (2012, 2 July). We're Not Here for Your Inspiration. Retrieved 25 August, 2012, from www.abc.net.au/rampup/articles/2012/07/02/3537035.htm

YouTube. (2014). About YouTube. Retrieved 3 March, 2014, from http://www.youtube.com/yt/about/en-GB/

Yuan, D. (1996). The Celebrity Freak: Michael Jackson's 'Grotesque Glory'. In R. Garland-Thomson (ed.), *Freakery: Cultural Sectacles of the Extraordinary Body* (pp. 368–84). New York and London: New York University Press.

Zara, C. (2014, 2 January). American Girl Responds To Melissa Shang, Who Wants A 'Girl Of The Year' Doll With A Disability. Retrieved 26 January, 2014, from http://www.ibtimes.com/american-girl-responds-melissa-shang-who-wants-girl-year-doll-disability-1525416

Zeisler, A. (2008). *Feminism and Pop Culture.* Berkley: Seal Press.

Zhang, L., and Haller, B. (2013). Consuming Image: How Mass Media Impact the Identity of People with Disabilities. *Communication Quarterly, 61*(3), 319–34. doi: 10.1080/01463373.2013.776988

Žižek, S. (2010, 4 March). Avatar: Return of the natives. Retrieved 9 January, 2014, from http://www.newstatesman.com/film/2010/03/avatar-reality-love-couple-sex

Filmography

21 Jump Street (1987–1991), 20th Century Fox Television, USA

A Nightmare on Elm Street (1984), Wes Craven, USA

Ally McBeal (1997–2002), Fox, USA

America's Next Top Model (2003–), 10 by 10 Entertainment, Pottle Productions, Ty Ty Baby Productions, USA.

Australia's Got Talent (2007–), FremantleMedia Australia, Australia

Avatar (2010), James Cameron, USA

Beverly Hills 90210 (1990–2000), 90210 Productions, USA

Beverly Hills 90210 (2008–2013), CBS Productions, USA

Big Brother (2000–), Bazal, Brighter Pictures, Channel 4 Television Corporation, USA

The Bionic Woman (1976–1978), Harve Bennett Productions, USA

Bionic Woman (2007–), NBC, USA

Blade Runner (1982), Ridley Scott, USA

Born on the Fourth July (1989), Oliver Stone, USA

Breaking Bad (2008–2013), High Bridge Productions, Gran Via Productions, Sony Pictures Television, USA.

Britain's Got Talent (2005–), FremantleMedia, UK

Britain's Missing Top Model (2008), British Broadcasting Corporation (BBC), UK

Charlie's Angels (1976–1981), Screen Gems Network, USA

Coming Home (1978), Hal Ashby, USA

CSI: Crime Scene Investigation (2000–), Alliance Atlantis Communications, CBS Paramount Network Television, CBS Productions, USA.

Dumb and Dumber (1994), Peter Farrelly, Bobby Farrelly, USA

Extreme Makeover: Home Edition (2003), ABC, USA

Fame (1980), Alan Parker, USA

Firefly (2002–2003), Mutant Enemy, USA

Flashdance (1983), Adrian Lyne, USA

Friday Night Lights (2006–2011), Imagine Television, Film 44, NBC Universal Television, USA.

Game of Thrones (2011–), HBO, USA

Gattaca (1997), Andrew Niccol, USA

Glee (2009–), Brad Falchuk Teley-Vision, Ryan Murphy Productions, 20th Century Fox Television, USA.

Halloween (1978), John Carpenter, USA

Hannibal (2013–), Dino De Laurentiis Company, Living Dead Guy Productions, Gaumont International Television, USA.

Idol (2002–), Fremantle Media North America, Fremantle Media, 19 Television, USA.

James May Toy Stories (2009), Blockhead and May, UK

Life's Too Short (2011–), British Broadcasting Corporation (BBC), Home Box Office (HBO), Backlash Productions, UK.

Little People Big World (2006–), Gay Rosenthal Productions, USA

Lost (2004–2010), Bad Robot, USA

Masterchef (2010–), One Potato Two Potato, USA

Me, Myself and Irene (2000), Peter Farrelly, Bobby Farrelly, USA

Metropolis (1927), Fritz Lang, Germany

Million Dollar Baby (2004), Clint Eastwood, USA

Murderball (2005), Henry Alex Rubin, Dana Adam Shapiro, USA

My Gimpy Life (2011–), Dracogen, Rolling Person Productions, USA.

Parenthood (2010–), True Jack Productions, Imagine Television, Universal Media Studios, USA.

Project Runway (2004–), Bravo Cable, Bunim-Murray Productions (BMP), Full Picture, USA.

Push Girls (2012–), Gay Rosenthal Productions, USA.

Robocop (1987), Paul Verhoeven, USA

Serenity (2005), Joss Whedon, USA

Shrek (2001), Andrew Adamson, Vicky Jenson, USA

Star Trek (1966–1969), Desilu Productions, USA

Star Trek (2009), J.J. Abrams, USA

Star Trek: The Next Generation (1987–1994), Paramount Television, USA

Star Wars (1977), George Lucas, USA

Stuck on You (2003), Peter Farrelly, Bobby Farrelly, USA

Take a Seat: Sharing a Ride Across America (2011), Encompass Films, USA

Texas Chainsaw Massacre (1974), Vortex, USA

The Big Bang Theory (2007–), Chuck Lorre Productions, USA

The Cabinet of Dr. Caligari (1920), Robert Wiene, Germany

The Fake Beggar (1898), Thomas Edison, USA.

The Fast and the Furious (2001), Rob Cohen, USA

The Guild (2007–), RobotKittenGigglebus Entertainment, USA

The Last Leg (2012–), Open Mike Productions, UK

The Six Million Dollar Man (1974–1978), Harve Bennett Productions, USA

The Sopranos (1999–2007), HBO, USA

The Specials (2009), KADA Media Limited, UK

The Terminator (1984), James Cameron, USA

The Voice (2011–), NBC, USA

The Waterdance (1992), Neal Jimenez, Michael Steinberg, USA

The West Wing (1999–2006), John Wells Productions, Warner Bros Television, USA.

The X Factor (2004–), ITV, UK

There's Something About Mary (1998), Bobby Farrelly, Peter Farrelly, USA

Top of the Pops (1964–2012), BBC, UK

Twin Peaks (1990–1991), Lynch/Frost Productions, USA

Unbreakable (2000), M. Night Shyamalan, USA

Weeds (2005–2010), Lionsgate Television, USA

X-Men (2000), Bryan Singer, USA

Index

Note: References to figures are in **bold**.

For Product Safety Concerns and Information please contact our EU
representative GPSR@taylorandfrancis.com
Taylor & Francis Verlag GmbH, Kaufingerstraße 24, 80331 München, Germany

www.ingramcontent.com/pod-product-compliance
Ingram Content Group UK Ltd.
Pitfield, Milton Keynes, MK11 3LW, UK
UKHW020954180425
457613UK00019B/673

9 780367 669003